VOICES *of*
CANCER

What We Really Want, What We Really Need

Insights for Patients and the People Supporting Them

LYNDA
WOLTERS

www.mascotbooks.com

VOICES *of* CANCER

Cover portraits by Chris Taylor
facebook.com/chrisarttaylor
Instagram: @artistchris

Author photo on dust jacket by Taylor Humby, humbyart.com

The portraits on the cover of this book depict actual people who have been diagnosed with cancer. Their names are, from left to right and top to bottom: Chris Taylor, Nancy Beth, Vicky Wallace Stephens, Shannon Boven Glorioso, Jay Carter, Louis Chinn, Angela Crawford Perez, Debra Guinn Donatti, Kathy Ilk Trujillo, Joel Israel, Gail Fay, Jessica Gripentrog, Nancy Miller, Brandi Cash, Bradley Glassel, Mark Biron, Lynda Wolters, Kevin McGee, Laura DiGiambattista, Sabine Schawb

For more information, please contact:
Mascot Books
620 Herndon Parkway #320
Herndon, VA 20170
info@mascotbooks.com

Library of Congress Control Number: 2019905017

CPSIA Code: PRFRE0719A
ISBN-13: 978-1-64543-039-1

Printed in Canada

It goes without saying that this book would never have happened if it weren't for all my newfound friends in the cancer world, some of whom we have lost. All the people who were so open, honest, and willing to talk with me: you made this happen and this is for you.

I would also like to thank all the caregivers, friends, and loved ones who stick by us while we are sick; to you all goes a special thank you—without you we may not be here.

CONTENTS

PART TWO: Surviving Treatment—*the pain, emotional wreckage, debilitation, and the struggle to keep a grip on and maintain mental health.*

PART THREE: Forward into the New Normal—*once you have faced what could kill you, there's no going back.*

PART FOUR: Life Is Short ... for Everyone—
*choosing to live the rest of your life with
however much time you have left.*

PREFACE
My "Cancer Shift"

I WAS A NON-CANCER PATIENT once, standing on the outside of this horrific disease with my rose-colored glasses, dreaming of the perfect ending to my amazing, fun-filled life. I was going to live to eighty-five or so, have stylish silver hair, and wear old-lady polyester pants and colorful blouses (tucking a tissue up my sleeve like my grandmother used to do) and reading glasses that would perch at the end of my nose or hang from a delicate chain around my neck. I had my future retirement all planned out: travel, adventure, activities, grandchildren. And when the time came, I was going to pass away in my sleep. Nothing drawn-out, no pain; just put my head on the pillow one night, and *poof*! Gone.

My truth, however, is that I will never see any of that. That dream belonged to the person I was before my "cancer shift."

Before my diagnosis, I had only known a couple of people close to me who had cancer: my first cousin, Joni, and her mother, Aunt Ina. Of course, a friend of a friend or a parent of a friend got cancer, and, while I felt sad for them, cried with them, and sometimes attended a funeral for a friend's loved one, I was never on the frontline of the disease. I was sheltered, naïve, and unknowingly selfish.

I thought I did right by these people at the time. In my take on the world, no one would purposefully be rude, mean, or hurtful to someone who was sick, and I was no exception. However, since becoming a cancer patient, I have learned that I, like so many others, have been inadvertently hurtful to ill people whom I cared for and loved.

My aunt succumbed to the disease within a few years of her diagnosis. My cousin Joni survived. I love Joni like a sister, yet I shamefully failed her during her treatment. Not once did I visit her. Instead, I would check in with other family members to ask how Joni was doing. I would tell them, "Let Joni know I'm thinking of her, I'm here for her, and she can call me if she needs anything." Of course, she never called and, therefore, I assumed she didn't need anything.

Following Joni's illness, Aunt Ina was diagnosed with metastatic breast cancer. I visited my aunt often during her illness, driving the same distance that was seemingly too far when Joni was sick. I would drive the two hours to sit by her side, hold her hand in the hospital, and comfort both her and my mother, who had become one of her caregivers. I knew I needed to be present for them both, regardless of my own inconvenience. I am grateful beyond words that I made Aunt Ina a priority.

But I now know I failed Joni. I was too busy with my life, my children, and my job—too distracted with the noise of my world to put myself and my issues on hold long enough to drive the mere two hours to sit with and comfort Joni, hold her hand, bring her dinner, or clean her toilet. I am ashamed to say I found out long after Joni was in remission that she suffered alone during most of her illness … and her toilet wasn't cleaned for a year. She was too weak and too sick to take care of everyday chores herself. By not reaching out for help, she not only suffered alone through her illness but also had to endure an unclean toilet. Understand that this is common among cancer patients—we will not ask for assistance. Maybe it's simply human nature, pride, or denial that prevents us from admitting we're unable to do things for ourselves.

Years later, during my own battle with cancer, I reached out to Joni and apologized for not being present when she needed me the most. She was most gracious, explaining that I didn't need to apologize: "Sweetie, people just don't know what to say or do when someone has cancer." She readily forgave me for my dereliction of duty, and I swore I would never be that person again.

I had learned through my sheer naïveté with Joni's battle that speaking the words were not enough; I needed to not just say I was available, I needed to be *present*—to take the initiative and reach out with a specific offer, rather than burden the one battling the disease with one more thing to do. Better yet, I learned to take action without asking, putting into play the mantra: *Move forward then beg for forgiveness.*

It was only when I was diagnosed that I truly understood the full extent of the need for support, both for the patient and the caregiver. Emotional support is a necessary and vital component to a person's overall sense of well-being. This couldn't be truer in the face of a cancer diagnosis.

Like Joni, I too had to forgive the people I felt had abandoned me during my illness. I still carry the scars inflicted by friends and family who "didn't want to bother me" while I was sick, or figured I had enough people around and thought it best to wait until later to come see me. If they only knew the hours and days I spent without anyone by my side—alone, sad, and scared.

Joni reached out to me several times during my treatment. She overcame the wound I inflicted on her years earlier and gave me her time, showing she cared about me and loved me and that I mattered. She taught me a valuable lesson with her grace.

Cancer itself was a powerful teacher too. It taught me to be more in touch with others, to be more empathetic, and to be *present*—to see life through a different perspective with more clarity about self and others, to appreciate the little things, like squirrels and raindrops, and to live with less judgment and more smiles, more happy tears, and more love.

While I never wanted this diagnosis, I would never change what I have gained from my experience. What I offer to you is a glimpse into the minds and hearts of people with the disease so that you may understand their needs and feelings better. I also offer some ideas for what to say to them, what not to say to them, and how they want to be treated.

Cancer is terrifying to the patient and to the people around them. It is touching people every day and truly is a part of life. You can support your loved ones who suffer with it by reaching out to them with the small things that matter.

My Calling to Write This Book

I HAVE ALWAYS BEEN BLESSED with the gift of gab. My parents told me that when I was little, I would talk to anything; they once gave me a spoon with which I apparently carried on a lengthy one-sided conversation. In my defense, I was only two years old.

Growing up, my chattiness would sometimes get me in trouble, usually in the classroom. Most of the time, my gregarious personality meant that whomever I met for the first time did not remain a stranger for long, an attribute I appreciate. Having cancer has been an incredibly interesting way for me to put my gabby gift to use.

At the request of my husband, to avoid being forced to constantly repeat news of my treatment, I started an online journal to keep my friends and family up to date. This journal was initially rather clinical. I was reserved and cautious about what I wrote, not wanting to get too personal or too graphic. However, as time went on, I became more open and raw about my thoughts and feelings and what my body was really going through. In fact, people appreciated my genuineness when I wrote about having chronic diarrhea or being so irritated with my doctor that I walked out of an appointment.

My journal had a very loyal following that included complete strangers who were turned on to my journal by friends who thought they may benefit from my writing. I once met a lady at a football game who introduced herself and told me that she had read part of my journal while her daughter was going through breast cancer. She said my story of feeling abandoned by my mother during my treatment resonated with her, and she realized she was doing the same thing to her daughter. Through her tears she told me that because of my journal, she stepped up. She started going with her daughter to every appointment and treatment, and she had become one of her daughter's biggest supporters.

To meet people like this, to hear others gush about how grateful they were for my open dialogue and read comments of the journal's followers, was amazing. It was a huge encouragement for me to continue penning my journey. It's pretty hard to not feel compelled to continue when people tell you that they better understood what their loved one was going through in their cancer journey by reading my stories. I was humbled and inspired.

I began carrying around a small notebook and writing down things I heard as I was going through my treatment: snippets of conversations in waiting rooms and answers to questions I would ask other patients. I compiled these statements and began to realize there was a connection. I discovered that no matter who the patient was, where they came from, their background, their age (I only interacted with adults), or their beliefs, everyone felt the same: no one outside of another cancer patient really understood what they were going through.

Everyone had feelings of being alone and misunderstood—it seemed a universal issue. While supporters were doing the best they could, they often missed the mark when it came to understanding what the patients needed to hear, how they wanted to be taken care of, and what things they thought about.

There was also, I found, another consistent theme. Those who were facing a life-altering, perhaps terminal diagnosis had a new, very clear sense of perspective regarding life; they had a *cancer shift*.

I was encouraged by dozens of people, including doctors, nurses, patients, and caregivers, to write about the tough subjects relating to cancer. The inner thoughts we cancer patients do not readily share: the fear, the twisted humor, the newfound insight following the acceptance of the diagnosis, and the wish for others to appreciate the beauty that comes when clarity and perspective move together in the right direction.

That shift is simple: *life is fabulous!*

I began first with a cleansing memoir of my journey, which is complete and lying on the floor of my home office. There it will stay until I determine if it will be something for my family to read when I am gone, or perhaps tinder for a good fire before I pass.

It was just before my second "cancer-versary," while attending *Epic Experience*, a camp for adult cancer survivors in Colorado, when I had a clarity shift of my own and realized what I felt drawn to write about. Those who attended the camp were lightheartedly dubbed "Big-Girl Panties" (as in, "it's time to pull up your big-girl panties"); I love them all to the moon and back. It was from many of those other campers that I garnered much of the insight for this project. They were all so open, so honest, so genuine, and so willing to talk about subjects I threw their way.

During that week of self-discovery and self-actualization, I had found a way to put my knowledge of and association with this heinous disease to good use. Perhaps I could help enlighten those on the outside of cancer to better understand what it is like to be on the inside.

My Faith and My Diagnosis

I WASN'T BORN INTO A religion nor do I have a religious family; nevertheless, my personal faith runs deep. My dad was a ministry school dropout who didn't become a parishioner again for nearly fifty years. He must have had some personal issues with God to work through, but I will never know. My mom had a nonreligious upbringing, and her parents neither professed a belief nor declined one. However, I started attending church when I was five years old; I was simply drawn to it. After experiencing several different churches in my little hometown, I found Catholicism and was baptized at the age of twelve.

I was a devout young Catholic, participating weekly in confessing my sins and taking communion. When I moved out on my own, I began attending Mass in the morning and often at noon, as well as weekly Sunday Mass, and I thrived with the sense of control religion brought to my life. I knew just when to genuflect and do the sign of the cross and the stability of the rituals brought me great peace and comfort.

In my mid-twenties, my belief in religion crumbled. After six years and two children, my first marriage failed. I had stopped going to church through this chaotic time and was in spiritual turmoil. I needed to come back to my safe place, my home—church. I walked into the confessional, knelt down, and with the sign of the cross said to the priest behind the curtain, "Bless me, Father, for I have sinned. It has been quite some time since my last confession, and since then I have committed many sins." My head was bowed in shame. After confessing my sins to the priest, including remarrying, I was informed that without an annulment, the Church believed my second marriage was not valid. To them, I was living in sin and would no longer be allowed to receive the sacrament of Holy Communion. I was essentially excommunicated as being adulterous for remarrying without having an annulment. Now I was nothing but a harlot in the eyes of the Church. This was the end of my Catholic days.

I lost my religion, and my faith was shaken. I then spent many years avoiding God, embarrassed and ashamed that my life had turned into one marriage after another, when years earlier I had been so full of the Spirit that I once (albeit fleetingly) thought of becoming a nun. I was spiritually spiraling and losing control in my personal life.

During my days as a Catholic, I had never read or studied the Bible, only hearing snippets during Mass about the mysterious Matthew, Mark, Luke, and John who penned the Gospels in the Good Book. It wasn't until my Catholic doors were closed that I picked up a Bible to fill the void of my lost religious home. I began a habit of reading several pages every morning, a habit I would never quit.

Through the years, I have read the Bible's pages many times, with the exception of Revelation. I am afraid of that book because surely it will tell me I am to be sentenced to an eternity in some horrible place filled with screaming demons as a result of my unforgivable sins. My early religious teaching and guilt haunt me and keep me from finishing the Good Book. I am hopeful, however, that God will somehow spare me from damnation.

I learned through my morning readings that religion and faith are two separate and distinct matters. The former comprises the rules and prescriptions resulting from mankind's interpretation of the Bible, the latter being the belief that there is something bigger, greater, and divine beyond this earthly life. Faith I would hang on to; religion I would let go.

I share this because my faith in Heaven and God would be tested again at great lengths a few decades later. For many people living with cancer, a new or expanded perspective on faith or a higher power is, I believe, a major part of the cancer shift.

Shift Closer to Cancer

UNLESS YOU ARE A CANCER survivor or current sufferer, you will not experience the kind of cancer shift I and others like me have experienced. However, you can still shift closer to understanding what it means to live with cancer, and it is my aim in this book to help you do that.

I have done my best to capture many different perspectives, personalities, and insights from those whose cancer journeys are similar to and completely different from mine. I have talked with those who were diagnosed as stage 1 through stage 4. I have spent time with people in the healthcare field, questioning their perception of cancer and its ripple effect, and I have tried to cover some of the most difficult subjects.

My hope is that, by the end of the book, you will feel better equipped to interact with and support a cancer patient. Along the way, I also hope you will benefit from some of the clarity I and others have gained through our diagnoses about what is important in your own life.

PART ONE
Initial Reactions

*What is in the hearts and minds of many cancer patients
and what those around them need to understand.*

THE PATIENT

Time to Pull Up the Big-Girl Panties

Diagnosis shock and denial, confusion, and disbelief.

IF YOU ADOPT A REALISTIC/PESSIMISTIC VIEW, we are all dying from the minute we are born. But let's be honest, does anyone really think that way?

I have cancer, and I am dying.

I was diagnosed with terminal stage 4 non-Hodgkin mantle cell lymphoma three weeks after I turned forty-nine. Like everyone else, this was the last thing I ever expected to happen to me. After all, wasn't I the epitome of health? I ate right, considered kale a food group long before it was catapulted to the forefront of the superfood category, didn't drink, only smoked a little (don't we all lose our minds a little bit in our teenage years?), never did drugs, and exercised every weekday morning. For fun, several evenings per week, I would ballroom and swing dance. I was an outdoor fanatic of rafting, hiking, and all things that involved being out in the sun. I was one of the healthiest people I knew.

I have talked to many dozens of cancer patients and have learned that I am not alone in being a pre-cancer health nut; many of them felt they too were some of the healthiest people they knew prior to being diagnosed. And even the patients I spoke with who weren't necessarily health freaks never expected to get cancer.

There are those who get cancer and people think they should not be surprised—for example, a forty-pack-per-year smoker who gets lung cancer. However, no matter who you are, the lifestyle you lead, or where you are in your journey of life, it is still a complete and utter shock to hear the most dreaded three words, "You have cancer." The response is always, "I have what?! Are you kidding me?"

My diagnosis was no different. I was in absolute shock when those three fateful words were spoken to me. Yes, I had been tired, exhausted actually, but I chalked these issues up to dealing with the stress of my dad's recent passing. I would continue to use his death as the rationalization for my lymph nodes popping out the side of my neck two weeks after he passed. Certainly my new Frankenstein look could be attributed to stress, I kept hearing myself say. I had started losing weight, "Just a couple pounds," I told myself. I had difficulty eating and had taken to napping during the day. Again, couldn't all this be related to the stress of losing Dad? *Of course it could.*

When my husband, Jody, and I were in the doctor's office awaiting what we hoped were answers to my declining health, we had already done our own research. Well, in all actuality, I did the research. Jody was less than enthusiastic about information I gathered from "doctors" on WebMD and Google, and would get a bit snippy with me as I continually droned on about the type of cancer I was convinced I had.

He would say to me, "Why do you do this to yourself?" after my long hours of research and self-diagnosing.

"I need to know what is going on with me," I replied, continuing entering phrases into the search bar, looking for a connection to my symptoms: *constant throat clearing, weight loss, and fatigue. What are the symptoms of cancer? What are the symptoms of thyroid disease?*

My symptoms always led me back to one of two things: thyroid disease, which included thyroid cancer and non-Hodgkin lymphoma. Doctor Google and Doctor WebMD both came back with: *"Feelings of fatigue, generalized malaise, weight loss, and night sweats can be signs of lymphoma."* I did *not* have night sweats, so I would tell myself, "I certainly can't have lymphoma." Although I *sensed* I did.

I was stuck in my own crazy cycle going back and forth between thyroid issues and lymphoma, praying not to have the latter. I had convinced myself that having a thyroid issue of any kind, including cancer, would be the better option of the two that I was sure I was facing. I actually started praying that it was thyroid cancer. *After all,* I thought, *with medication you can live without your thyroid.*

In the couple of weeks prior to my diagnosis, I had a battery of tests, including a CT scan of my head and neck, a thyroid ultrasound followed by a fine-needle biopsy, and then a core biopsy. One of my Frankenstein lymph nodes was biopsied, and I had a PET scan. I made the newbie mistake of ordering and trying to interpret some of my records prior to the scheduled follow-up with my doctor.

I became fixated on research, trying to correlate what I thought my results said to what I was finding online, and I only had my husband to discuss my findings with. Unfortunately for him. He was my only sounding board, as I had refused to tell my children, my mother, or my friends about any of this, explaining, "I don't want to put any stress on them until I know something certain."

When the day came for Jody and me to hear the news about whether or not my feelings of fatigue and throat tightening were all in my head, perhaps related to generalized anxiety or something more ominous like cancer, we were as prepared as possible in our own way: I with my arsenal of research under my belt and questions in my notepad, and Jody with his head in the sand of denial, hoping this was all a manifestation of symptoms due to the stress of my father's passing.

When the doctor walked in the room, followed by the physician's assistant and the nurse, Jody and I both knew this was not a good sign. When do three providers come into an exam room? Only when there is bad news to deliver. Without so much as a greeting, the doctor sat down on the little round stool, clasped his hands in his lap, took an audible breath and said in a very somber tone, "You have B cell lymphoma, suggestive of mantle cell. I'm sorry."

Without a pause, perhaps to skate past what he had just said, or perhaps because he didn't want the full weight of his words to cause hysteria, he continued talking about tests and plans, specialists, and treatment. What I heard, however, was, "Wah-wah, wah-wah." His lips were moving, but I was still trying to comprehend what he had just said, and I could not make sense of any other words. I was suffering with what a fellow cancer patient called the Charlie Brown Syndrome. The teacher keeps talking, but all Charlie Brown hears is "Wah-wah, wah-wah."

"Wait, what?" I said to the doctor, as I held up my hand to stop him, "What about thyroid cancer?"

"You don't have thyroid cancer, you have lymphoma," he said patiently.

"But I thought the cancer was in my thyroid. All the tests—I read the reports, I researched everything—"

"The cancer is in your blood, in your lymph nodes, and it has spread to your thyroid," he explained. "I am sorry, but there is nothing I can do to help you. I need to refer you to a hematology oncologist, a blood cancer specialist."

The reality of the word *oncologist* hit hard. I looked at my husband, sitting in the corner of the room, his jaw slightly open and his eyes full of tears ready to fall. "What is he talking about?" I asked in a whisper, oblivious to the others in the room. Unable to utter a word, Jody could do no more than sit in his chair and stare at me in disbelief.

The next few weeks were spent having more tests, scans, biopsies, ultrasounds, and numerous doctor visits who confirmed what was already suspected: I did, in fact, have stage 4 non-Hodgkin lymphoma (NHL). The specific type of NHL was known as mantle cell lymphoma (MCL). By the time of my diagnosis, the cancer had spread to the lymph nodes in my neck, axilla (armpit), and groin. It had settled heavily in my thyroid and was throughout my gastrointestinal tract from "tip to stern," and in my bones. All of my mystery symptoms had suddenly been validated.

MCL is a very rare strain of NHL. Only 5 percent of people with NHL have mantle cell. But an even more distressing fact I learned was that of those who get MCL, three-quarters are men over sixty. *Really?* I was a forty-nine-year-old female. My youngest son would later say to me, "Mom, you not only drew the short straw, you drew the *shortest* straw."

On the silent ride down in the elevator from the doctor's office that first day of my diagnosis, I came to a very clear decision—my first *cancer shift*. I was going to go through this journey with openness, honesty, and hopefully grace. Right then and there, I turned to my husband of only one year and said, "You don't have to do this. You don't have to stay."

Jody was appalled by my statement. "What are you talking about?" he asked me with tears rolling down his cheeks, still stunned by the words from the doctor.

"You didn't sign up for this." I told him. "Look," I said, "No one would blame you if you just walked away now. I am giving you that out. Honestly, I would understand if you just left. But if you do leave you have to do it now. You can't do it later or you will just be looked at as the jerk who left his dying wife."

We stood in the heat of the sun outside the doctor's office, looking at each other, both shocked by the results of the past several weeks, and he said to me, "I'm not going anywhere. I love you."

"Okay," I said, "but you have to stay now. You can't leave me."

"I won't," Jody said, "but you can't push me away either."

His resolve would be tested sooner than we thought because, after the initial round of tests, came the sobering revelation from my oncologist who informed me—out of the blue—that there was no cure for this type of cancer. He not only told me it was terminal but also that the average life expectancy, once diagnosed at this stage, was five years. At that moment, I was not prepared for such news, so once more I fell back into the Charlie Brown Syndrome, hearing only, "Wah-wah, wah-wah."

Neither my husband and I, nor my life, would ever be the same again. It was time to pull up those big-girl panties and fight for my life.

I'm Not Mad at God

Faith is in your control and fate is a matter of circumstance.

PEOPLE ARE SURPRISED WHEN I tell them I am not angry at God for my diagnosis; some people are even surprised when I tell them I still have faith. I am a firm believer that we all have our lot in life and, for whatever reason, being diagnosed with a terminal illness is mine.

I do not look at my diagnosis as a punishment; I am not a bad person. Even if I were, cancer is not something anyone deserves. My diagnosis just _is_.

"But why _you?_" my dear friend Gricelda asked me at the beginning of my treatment.

"Why not me?" I asked her back. I reminded her none of us are guaranteed anything, including freedom from illness. I also told Gricelda that I would rather be the one going through this than a young mother, like her, who hasn't finished raising her babies.

I have been blessed throughout my life and still am. I was able to successfully raise my sons and lead a rich life filled with happiness, love, and laughter. I still feel that way. Being sick did not take those things away; it only enhanced their specialness.

Susan, a breast cancer survivor, said about her journey, "Cancer can change your body, and it can surely take your body away, but it _can't_ have your spirit."

For reasons unknown to me, God has chosen me to go through this, and I want to do it with grace. I choose not to be bitter and angry because I feel there is a bigger message that I am supposed to share beyond the fact that I have cancer.

Oh, don't misunderstand and think that I have never had words with God about my cancer; in fact, there have been times when I have truly cried out in anger, pain, and desperation. My journey has been filled with immense suffering and agony caused by my joints and bones, and there have been times I've begged God for relief and waited for months without any response.

One particularly excruciatingly painful morning, I found myself sitting on the floor of my shower, my body wracked with sobs, alone in my head, asking the questions that surely crosses everyone's mind who has a similar diagnosis: "Why me, God?" Other times I would cry out loud, "Please help me, God."

In the end, relief always came, but sometimes I failed to see that until I looked back and realized that eventually the pain or the frustration would stop; it just wasn't always in the time frame I wanted.

My life during the days of pain was little more than an existence. Sometimes I hurt so bad that I am surprised I survived. When the pain would dissipate, I would be overjoyed and grateful for the relief. I came to understand that a good day was as simple as one without pain.

It is during my times of great suffering, of feeling alone and scared, that I find my deepest sense of faith—when I actually *feel* the presence of something much greater than me, encouraging me to *take the next right step*. For me, it is faith that keeps me going; faith that there is a purpose for everything and faith that there is something better waiting for me.

When I am not well, I experience much greater spiritual clarity. At my sickest moment, while going through my third round of chemotherapy, I felt I was standing on the precipice between continuing to fight and letting go, but I *knew* I had a choice; I could either take the next breath or be done, and in that moment of clarity, I had never felt so much peace. The calmness that surrounded that moment is hard to describe. I had no thoughts, no pain, no fear, just a *sense* that no matter which way I decided to go, it was going to be all right. It was at that moment that all the noise vanished and I learned that I was no longer afraid of dying.

It was also at this moment that I first experienced what is meant by "be still and listen." This doesn't necessarily mean that you will be literally tapped on the shoulder and hear someone; it simply means that when you stop trying to get past your current state and accept where you are *now*, there is a sense of contentment, of understanding.

Prayers Are Not for Everyone

I SPEND A GOOD DEAL of time in prayer, including praying for myself, for healing and grace. I can see how easy it could be to become bitter and hateful, blaming God and wondering why. I made a conscious decision to continue to remain grateful for my blessings, to thank God for the good days, and to keep my wrestling with Him to a minimum.

God has been faithful to me and has already answered my biggest prayer, that He not take me home until after my boys were raised. As a single mom, I always asked God that whatever He had in store for me to please keep it at bay until my boys were grown. He gave me an additional six years thereafter before I was diagnosed. That is a blessing. My prayers were answered, and I remind myself to keep that gratitude in the forefront of my mind while walking through my cancer journey.

Since my diagnosis, I have met all types of people from all walks of life, including those with a belief in God and those without, as well as those somewhere in between. I learned a good lesson from Mary Margaret, who is a Catholic turned agnostic. She told me it is troubling, almost burdensome, when people tell her they will pray for her. She explained that while she generally just thanks the person and goes on her way, she wishes that people would not assume just because she has cancer that she has an automatic belief in God.

Voices on Prayer

PEOPLE WITH AN AGNOSTIC VIEW of the beyond feel more comfortable hearing, "I will keep you in my thoughts." And Mary Margaret, like all of us, would like to hear that good vibes are being sent her way.

Brad also considers himself an untraditional believer. He feels that while "I'll pray for you" is better than a "do good" sentiment, it might be nice to add an "I care for you" type of statement.

Kate suggests offering: "I will be sending you light," and Denise adds to that sentiment with: "Sending you love and light."

Eric's suggestion is to offer something tangible in the place of a prayer; perhaps to pick up the cancer sufferers' children for them one day or to make them dinner.

Jordan says that while he realizes offering prayer is meant to convey something positive, it is his experience that it tends to lean more toward, "I am going to talk about being positive to you instead of actually doing or saying anything meaningful." When he told me this, he was quick to point out that he does not want to demean an obvious kind wish, but the phrase "I will pray for you" feels impersonal and seems to be more about the speaker who wants to feel they are helping but for their own gratification, not his. Jordan would rather hear something intended to be uplifting to him, as an individual, than a recitation of a general cliché that satisfies the well-wisher's sense of obligation or guilt.

Eric suggested I listen to a podcast by an atheist who describes this scenario: "What do you say when a person offers prayers?" I found the podcast quite interesting and very informative. Essentially, I learned that if you know the person's religious affiliation or lack thereof, be considerate of it! If you don't know where they stand, it seems generally acceptable to say you will pray for them, but don't be offended if you are not met with a returned response of gratitude. Perhaps it is just better to say to acquaintances, "I will keep you in my thoughts."

It would seem, regardless of the belief system in place, that the people I spoke to have at least one thing in common regarding this subject: they all appreciate the well-wishes and will not turn them away. They believe that being a good person is paramount and putting out positivity is good karma and helpful to all.

I asked my friend, Mark, a former priest now battling brain cancer, for his opinion. He said, "If you look at history, there are many different prophets: Buddha, Mohammed, Jesus, and Martin Luther King Jr., just to name a few. I believe that, throughout history, these people have prophesied about a being that is gentler, more giving, and more loving and caring than us humans. We are all striving to be more like them, and that's the goal."

To that end, and with all good intentions, and without knowing your preferred religious stance, I wish you all love and light, positive vibes, and prayers of health. (I really did just say a prayer for everyone of faith reading this!)

THE NON-PATIENT

Relationships Change When Cancer Appears

*When your loved one has cancer, stepping up can be
difficult and stepping away can seem easier.*

When you get sick, you will be surprised by who steps up and
who steps away. I can honestly say I did not think this would apply
to me. I could not imagine that anyone in my family or circle of
friends would not be there for me. *Wrong!*

For the first four months after my diagnosis, my mom cried
literally every time I saw her. She avoided me and any conversation
dealing with my illness. She did not know the details of my care
or treatment and only went to one appointment with me, where
she sat in the waiting room with tears in her eyes that then flowed
throughout the entire appointment. She was not equipped to stand
by me, and I was not equipped to understand this.

My mom lives one mile from me and three miles from my clinic and hospital. She was capable, able, and unencumbered to support me but was too completely devastated and paralyzed by my diagnosis to do so. She only visited me a couple times during my week-long hospital stays. "I can't handle seeing you hooked up to all the tubes and machines," she told me. "I know I am a coward."

At one point, I sat with her and I did the crying. I poured out my heart, laying my feelings and justifications at her feet, explaining how I felt about her abandonment. She looked at me with tears rolling down her own cheeks and said the only thing she could: "I don't know what to say to you." I would hear those simple words repeated in nearly every circle of my life: family, friends, coworkers. Because people had no idea what to say to me, for me, or about me, they often avoided me instead.

As a result, I was quick to reach out to support groups and get involved in online chat rooms after my diagnosis. I would talk to anyone who had an ear and an extra minute. I started seeing a social worker through my clinic, and later a counselor, and built a support system of strangers that I could reach out to day or night. I figured my family and my husband would want to do the same thing.

Counseling for family was free at my cancer clinic, so it was something I not only suggested but also requested of my husband and mother. My two oldest children lived out of state, so this service could not benefit them, and my youngest was interning with a neuropsychologist at the time, so I figured he was covered.

My mother could not bring herself to go to counseling. Something always came up or she would promise to call them the next day. Regardless, it never happened.

Jody was no better. He point-blank said to me, "I don't have any questions, why do I need to go to counseling?"

In my newly diagnosed cancer mind, what I heard him say was, "I don't care enough to have any questions," or "My wife has a terminal illness, but I'm okay with it." This made me feel angry and abandoned. I felt as if I were alone on my own island. My mom didn't care enough to speak to me or a counselor, and my husband felt things were just fine the way they were. This made me crazy.

Voices on Counseling

I TOLD JODY ONE NIGHT while I was in the hospital, "I feel like I am in a life raft with holes in it, sharks circling, and you are on a white sandy beach under a palm tree. The sun is shining for you, you have a cocktail in your hand, and you are waving to me."

His response was, "I have to stay positive and not go down your negative rabbit hole."

Need I say that was not the right thing to say?

Jody and I went around and around about counseling. I would cry and plead for him to go, he would say, "Fine, you make the appointment, and I will go." But of course, I wanted *him* to make the appointment because that would show me he really wanted to do it, not just to pacify me.

I came to a point when I realized he simply did not think nor feel the same way I did. He was handling my diagnosis and his feelings differently, and that was going to have to be okay with me. I didn't have to like it, but worrying about him doing what I thought he should was taking too much energy from me, and I didn't have any to spare.

Kevin, who has a diagnosis of lymphoma, explained to me that my husband's behavior was natural and not anyone's fault.

"You just have cancer," Kevin said. "Just like me—I just have cancer. It's not your husband's fault, just as it's not my wife's fault: we just have cancer. And all the complaining you want to do to try to get your husband to counseling is not going to get him there. Men want to fix things, including things they didn't break. He can't fix you, so he doesn't feel he has anything to gain from counseling. It isn't because he doesn't love you; he just can't fix you." I appreciated the heartfelt lesson in male logic.

Kevin was right about Jody, but it took me nearly two years to understand that. Jody, as with most men, is a fixer. He can't fix me, so he wasn't going to go to counseling to talk about it because, in his mind, there was nothing to say. However, his choosing to not get counseling had nothing to do with how he felt about me. I had to learn to accept that.

I also had to figure out a way to accept the same thing regarding my mom. That was harder, however—she was my *mom*. She was my lifelong nurturer, my safe place through all my growing-up woes, and with my dad gone, she was the only person the little girl inside of me could run to. But she was unavailable, and I was crushed. I was asked during my treatment how my mom's absence made me feel. My response: "It makes me miss my dad."

My friends, while generally quite available for me, also had some rough times dealing with my diagnosis. They too didn't know what to say to me and, therefore, often avoided me.

They knew I had family in town, so they didn't want to step on any toes. But I wanted them stepping on toes. I wanted their frivolity and their water-cooler gossip that would make me laugh. I wanted them to distract me from my own life.

While going through treatment, I had lunch with a group of my closest friends. I asked them why they were so distant, and I learned they were uncomfortable and scared to say the wrong thing because they didn't want to upset me. This conversation prompted me to post the following in my blog, titled "A Letter from the Dying Girl."

If you are reading this, it is because you have been following along with my journey. It also means that we are friends, that somewhere along the way we have shared a part of each other's lives—a laugh, a story, a connection. Whether we have known each other for decades or have just met, we have a bond. We are in a relationship.

As we all know, relationships are not always easy, and this is one of those times. I will be starting the toughest part of my treatment, my inpatient chemotherapy. I know you are scared; I am too. And I know you don't always know what to say to me. I understand that as well. No one knows better than I the fear, the pain, the sickness, the diagnosis, and the prognosis.

Am I dying? Yes. Today? No. I have a terminal illness, and there is no cure at this time. Yes, I believe in miracles, but I am not holding out for one. This makes me sad, just like I am sure it does you. But in an odd way, I feel blessed by this knowledge because I feel it has given me a deeper understanding of what a relationship is and what is important in life.

A relationship does not mean that you only get the good. You also get the bumps, the long spans of time without communicating, and the words that hurt and leave scars. It also means being brave and courageous when the other person can't be. A relationship means stepping out of your comfort zone to say the words that are frightening, to have the conversations that you would rather avoid.

Right now, I need you. And I need you to understand that I cannot give you anything back at this time. Now is the time when you will have to be the giver in our relationship as I need your friendship and energy, your words, and your prayers. I will do my best to be available for you, but right now I can't make any promises.

Please don't be afraid to "bother" me. I want to be bothered with your phone call, text, or visit. It doesn't have to be much, just a quick touch to say, "I am here for you." And just like the old days, you can talk to me about anything. Trust me, I would rather hear about you, your work, your life, your kids, and your puppy's antics than I would about my sickness. I hear about that all day, every day.

I understand you will have questions, and it's okay to ask. I would rather you be honest and forthright than side-step the obvious. The only elephant in the room will be the one on your leash; you can leave him at the door.

I would rather see your face and the pain and fear in your eyes than to have you feel too unsure and awkward to see me. I am still the same me, the same girl you connected with and formed a relationship with; I am just sick now.

So, what do you say to the dying girl? Anything you want.

I am not alone with these tough-love issues. "Melanie" (I changed her name because I am hopeful the real-life mother-in-law of this person reads this passage one day), who suffers a chronic form of leukemia, has had to defend her diagnosis against her mother-in-law, Gloria (name changed), for years. Gloria seems to think that Melanie's cancer is not too difficult. "After all, you still have your hair!" she told Melanie one day. She has also had to endure comments for years about the fact that her chemotherapy regimen, which is in the form of daily or ever-other-day pills, is *easy*. "You have the easy cancer," Gloria has told her.

Melanie has tried in vain to get Gloria to understand that no cancer is easy, that she is just as sick as anyone with cancer, that her thoughts, feelings, and fears are just as real, valid, and overwhelming as anyone else's with a life-threatening disease. Melanie has had to *justify* her cancer.

Fortunately, Melanie has been taking baby steps to set boundaries regarding Gloria's cruel behavior, but her boundaries have been met with eye rolls and scoffs. In a sad twist of irony, Melanie's mother-in-law now has an extremely aggressive form of cancer, which will likely take her life in a few short months.

Melanie is devastated for a few reasons. She loves Gloria and understands how it feels to have cancer, but she also knows now that she will likely never get any resolution or amends regarding her mother-in-law's callous behavior. Melanie has chosen to take the high road and forego her desire to teach Gloria that her bad behavior is unacceptable. Rather, she now sits at Gloria's side and will hold her hand through her remaining treatments, being present for Gloria during her last days. I admire Melanie greatly and have learned from her example.

Tami, who has breast cancer and whose treatment included a double mastectomy, suffered at the hands of her entire family. They were supportive through her treatment and available during her surgeries, but four years later, they asked Tami when she is going to stop talking about and worrying about her cancer; after all, it *is* gone, they say to her.

Tami has set boundaries for herself regarding the insensitive behavior of her family, choosing to confide more in her friends who are fellow cancer sufferers when it comes to her ongoing anxiety surrounding her cancer. She has found a way to love her family while protecting herself.

I have come to realize that sometimes people, including those whom we love the most, may not have the words to say when someone they love is faced with a terminal illness. People tend to be afraid of cancer as it gives a finite face to life. Most people go around knowing one day they will die but not having a clue as to when. Those of us with a terminal illness have been given a probable timeline for our demise, and that is frightening. For those without the diagnosis, we are a reminder that they too will one day face their own mortality.

I learned that I needed to acknowledge the fear of my friends and family and give them permission to be just as scared as I am. I also learned that I need to forgive those who do not understand that what they do, and sometimes what they don't do, has the power to be hurtful and unwittingly destructive.

I too was an offender in many of these ways prior to being diagnosed. No one taught me how to behave or what to say to a sick person beyond the pleasantries of, "How are you?" and "I will keep you in my prayers." I guess somehow it was just expected that everyone simply knows what to do.

I have also learned that while my cancer is all about me, my relationships are not. Cancer takes its toll with a ripple effect, touching everyone around it. There is no right or wrong when it comes to dealing with its effects, but we need to be honest and openly communicate to bring the unspoken issues to the surface where they can be addressed.

My mother and I have a good relationship again. We have talked extensively about her absence during my treatment, and we have both come to terms with it. My open wounds are closed now, and the scars are fading. Time is precious—my mother is not getting any younger, and my days are limited. She and I now morbidly chuckle about which of us will finish the race first. We both hope the other loses.

Jody and I weathered the lack-of-counseling storm and have grown incredibly as a couple by confronting the issues surrounding my illness and communicating more. Through our differences, similarities were found; we each just wanted to be heard, we each needed to process in our own way, and we each needed to be allowed the safe space to do both.

I believe that no one is put in front of you by accident; there is a reason for it. And in ways big or small, each person will affect the other. You are either put in front of someone to teach them something or to learn a lesson from them. The lesson that my cancer diagnosis and I had to teach those around me was that they must not let their fear keep them from me. The lesson I had to learn was to practice grace with those who are afraid.

Intimacy and Cancer

When a loved one has a life-threatening illness, it changes everyone's perspectives in unexpected and sometimes far-reaching ways.

EVERYONE WANTS TO BE LOVED and to be wanted, and physical touch can be paramount to a healthy life. This can be in the form of a hug of reassurance, comfort or love, a handshake of greeting or for a job well done, or through the intimacy of a sexual relationship.

In my situation, emotional intimacy became a replacement for physical intimacy during my treatment. There were many things that would deter or derail any attempt at physicality, including pain, illness, nausea, vomiting, diarrhea, loss of self-image, worry over infection, and the list goes on. I was also told not to have intercourse for the first three days following my chemotherapy or to use a condom if I did. Apparently, the chemicals can be passed through bodily fluids. The fear of the possible transference of chemicals was also enough to curtail my husband's desire; I don't blame him for that.

From Jody's perspective, there was a special list of concerns from a spouse's perspective: fear of hurting me or causing an infection, misunderstanding my pain or emotional state, how to convince me that the physical differences in my body was *not* unattractive or noticeable or unsexy, and so on. Such worries are common to all spouses and partners.

I wanted a sex life during my treatment, regardless of how lofty the idea. My husband, however, was emotionally wrapped up in caring for me. All of my new maladies brought on by treatment overwhelmed him, so sex was not on his radar. For reasons of his own or for reasons he thought best for me, sex was just not realistic during my treatment, and this became a contentious issue for me.

I got frustrated and cried out, "Don't you want me anymore?" Jody would tell me he did, that he loved me and such, but what I meant was, "Don't you want *sex* with me anymore?"

It wasn't that I had a great need for it at that particular time or was even remotely turned on at any time during my treatment; I was just afraid of not having sex ever again. Maybe I thought this would be my last hoorah, or maybe I was worried that our new, eighteen month-old marriage would not survive without sex.

"I don't want to die without having sex again," I yelled at Jody one night. Looking back, I was completely out of my mind when I said this, as I was lying in my hospital bed receiving chemo. My husband was helpless. Even if screaming at him that I wanted sex had made him feel romantic, the setting was hardly conducive to acting upon it! I was simply an emotional wreck with a physical and/ or psychological need that could not be met.

I ended up in counseling to help me deal with several issues surrounding my cancer, including the shift in my physical relationship. Jody and I have survived my cancer thus far with our marriage intact, but many marriages fail. Research shows that at least 50 percent of couples break up during a cancer diagnosis.[1] This "partner abandonment" is because one partner or the other cannot handle the stress, the body changes, a new inability to have children, the financial pressure, the lack of sex, and so on.

The statistics also show that women who were told they had a serious illness are seven times more likely to be abandoned as men with similar health problems.[2] Studies show that women are more apt to stick it out if their partner is diagnosed with cancer, whereas men tend to leave. Being a caregiver seems to be less natural for men, and when they are forced to clean their spouse's wounds, bathe them, and generally take care of them, men feel more uncomfortable with these duties than women do. One cancer patient I spoke to stated that most people think of the marriage vow "in sickness and in health" applies at seventy or eighty years old when your spouse is in bed with pneumonia; the vow is not valid for a young spouse with a partner who is sick for months or years with cancer.

Voices on Broken Relationships

I HAVE CHOSEN NOT TO use the names of the patients I spoke with regarding this subject, as most of them are still with their partners, and I did not want to put their relationships at risk. I have also chosen not to delve at too great a length into this subject, as it is too vast and has a great many psychological components that I am not professionally qualified to address. Therefore, I have written an overview of the topic in order to put it out there for discussion. I wish you all positive communication with this subject.

Nearly everyone I spoke with admitted there was a change in their personal relationships once they were diagnosed. Some admitted that they or their significant other were completely turned off by the thought of sex: either one or both parties could not focus on anything other than how the patient looked or how they felt. However, some stated they had no issues whatsoever and life went on as normal regarding sex. I envy them. Interestingly, though, nearly all who stated that their sex life was fine were men with cancer.

I have met young men and women who lost their relationships

due to chemotherapy-induced sterility issues. This is heartbreaking because each of those survivors wanted children. Not only did they lose the ability to have their own children but they also lost their partner as well.

I have met women who, after having mastectomies, learned that their husbands—who would not have sex with them—had taken on another sexual partner. Whether or not this was because of the mastectomies is unknown; to the women, of course, it certainly felt too coincidental to not be a factor.

On the other hand, I know of men with cancer who purposefully pushed away a partner because they couldn't handle the idea of no longer pleasing them sexually after physical changes resulting from treatment or surgery.

I have listened to numerous stories about how single people intentionally stay single once diagnosed because they don't want to burden someone with the inevitable role of caregiver. Or even sadder, they wonder who could possibly want them now that they have a cancer diagnosis.

But not all the stories are sad. I must share, to the best of my memory, one of the most romantic love stories I know.

This happened with my cousin Joni during her cancer treatment. She was dragged to a casino by some coworkers just to get her out of the house. Joni was uncomfortable about going because she was not a gambler and, as she was in active treatment, felt and looked sick. She agreed to go, however, at the insistence of her friends. On the same day, a man named Brad, who also was not a gambler and was equally uncomfortable about being there, had been dragged to the same casino by a coworker. Brad saw Joni sitting with her friends and turned to his friend, telling him, "I'm going to marry that woman."

Brad made his way over to Joni and insisted they have dinner. Joni declined at first but ultimately spent time with Brad, learning that he was not only handsome but charming and had very similar interests in matters of importance to her. Brad, who lived in Nevada, began to travel to Idaho during Joni's treatments, sitting with her, caring for her, and helping her feel worthy of love during her most horrible days.

Brad and Joni's budding relationship grew and Brad proposed while Joni was still in treatment. Joni did her best to convince Brad that he should not marry her: "What about the finances?" she would say. Or "I can't thrust you into being a caregiver." But Brad didn't care. He loved her, and he was tired of being excluded in matters of her care because he was not a family member. He insisted, and she finally agreed. They have been married for more than twelve years.

Some people I spoke to have unfulfilling marriages and admitted that rather than leave their relationship, they have found a significant other to step into the role of sexual partner, replacing the missing component in their current relationship. Others simply do not think they will ever have the mindset to want a physical relationship ever again.

Unfortunately, several of the people told me they have divorced, separated, or moved on from their once monogamous relationships since diagnosis.

It did not matter who the person was—young, old, male, female, gay, or straight—no one was immune to the extreme stress cancer has on their physical relationship. How do you hold your relationship together through this insidious disease? From my experience, communication has been key. Pushing my kneejerk reaction of, "I want sex" to the back burner and learning to speak more rationally with my husband about my thoughts and feelings were of paramount importance. I also had to learn to accept the time frame of his own recovery from being my caregiver. It is important to be open and honest, understanding and kind, and communicate with love as the motivator. After all, there was likely once something special and uncomplicated with your sexual relationship prior to cancer.

The personal lesson I learned from this is that everything changes with cancer—*everything*. Life will never be the same again, even if on the smallest of levels, something will forever be different. There is no going back to who you once were, so embrace it and grow from it and with it. Find the new you in your new space and make it wonderful. If you seek out the good, you will find it, even in the darkest of situations, even if that means you are alone and without a partner or without physical intimacy. Find the ability to understand (even if you don't like it) that not everyone can handle the changes that occur from this disease. And remember life is precious and short. Be happy, be kind, and be the light for others that you want them to be for you.

Clichés, Buzz Words, and Being Positive

Honesty is the best approach—and some understanding of how cancer patients see their illness can help. Clichéd terms and thoughtless positives don't work.

IN OUR CURRENT CULTURE OF political correctness, we are all learning new ways to communicate with each other, embracing our differences, and finding ways to be inclusive without discrimination. It is why society no longer accepts offensive terms such as the "N-word," and why we have replaced gender biased terms, like "mailman" with "mail carrier." We changed our vocabulary because we became educated about how our words, while perhaps not meant to be disparaging or hurtful, were often just that out of sheer ignorance. If we have never walked in that person's shoes, never worn their skin tone or lived in their region, we may not know or understand what was offensive to them. Through years of becoming a more sensitive world, we are all learning how to communicate in a less derogatory manner. This, however, has fallen short when it comes to how we speak to people who have been given a devastating diagnosis. It is my contention that there are still some areas that need work; speaking of diagnoses is one of them.

Voices on Thoughtless Words

BE AWARE OF SOME COMMON irritating phrases.

"You look good, though." While a seemingly harmless thing to say, when the patient is going through treatment, they know they look different or ill but certainly not "good," at least in their eyes. Therefore, this statement can often feel more like an attempt to placate or avoid the obvious, which is not helpful. Rather than stating what feels like a little white lie to make the person with the illness feel better, it is more appreciated to hear something believable, such as, "It's good to see you. I can see you're going through a lot right now, and I am sure that is difficult for you." This puts the person first, and it is a respectful acknowledgment of the difference in appearance.

Vanity is not necessarily the issue here, but cancer changes everything and we know it: we feel it, we see it. Our skin changes tone, sometimes pale, ashen, yellow, or greenish. We get dark circles under our eyes and blemishes, boils, rashes, and herpes zosters (shingles) on our skin. We lose our hair, eyebrows, and eyelashes, as well as nose hair and pubic hair. There is weight gain and loss, atrophy of muscles, and once shapely bodies become misshapen with flab and cellulite from lack of exercise. The shape of our faces can change to a "moon face" due to steroids. Often, we have weird ports and PICC lines, tubes, drains, and bags of fluid showing out of our chest, neck, arms, and so on.

We patients see someone different looking back at us in the mirror, and we know you see it too. It's okay to be honest: we have enough mystery in our lives with our treatment and body changes, we don't need our friends and family adding to that layer of unknown with what feels like untruths.

"At least you got the good cancer." This one just blows me away, for many reasons. Before my diagnosis, while I was waiting for my results, I actually prayed that I had an "easy" cancer. What was I thinking? Is there such a thing? Regardless of the stage or the type, cancer is terrifying and ominous, and it will haunt you for the rest of your life. So, a good cancer? There is no such thing.

"I'm sorry." This is a tough one, and I have been known to use it myself when I didn't know what else to say. I am guessing that is why it is used by others as well. It seems to be unwelcome, however, because it is an easy catch-all phrase with no real meaning behind it. A child uses, "I'm sorry" to get out of trouble regardless of meaning it. "I'm sorry" is not an apology nor should it be used when you don't know what else to say—after all, my diagnosis is not your fault and you didn't do anything to be sorry about. Perhaps it would fall easier on the ears if "I'm sorry" is followed by "you have to go through this."

"That's life." When my friend Mark, who is battling brain cancer, told me this was one of his most-hated phrases after his diagnosis, I had no words. Really, who would say that to a cancer patient? I am thinking I would just walk away from that one and regroup, as I am not sure the speaker would even deserve a response.

"Bless your heart." This always makes me laugh because I can hear my friends Susan and Anastasia, both of whom have cancer, say this with a condescending twang: "Why, bless your heart, honey." (Imagine a hand on a hip and a downward tilt of the head, eyes peering over the tops of glasses.) Perhaps we just take the blessing and run with this one.

"Be strong." Is there any other choice?

"You got this." *Yes, I do have this; I have cancer. Thank you for reminding me*, runs through my head every time someone says this to me.

"Keep fighting." Refer to the "Be strong" comment above.

"This is just a season." Hmm, a season. So, this person thinks that cancer is a passing phase? Perhaps it is a blip in time that will soon be replaced by some different but equally awful *season* like typhoid or a ruptured appendix?

"Let me know if there is anything I can do." As mentioned earlier, this is a nice statement and makes the speaker feel better. But I guarantee it's not likely any cancer patient will call you, in part because we feel awkward showing vulnerability (aren't we all raised to take care of ourselves?). And our silence is also partly because we have absolutely no idea what it is we need until we actually need it. And then it is usually too late to reach out to anyone outside of our immediate caregiver. HINT: Proactivity definitely trumps passivity.

There is no perfect thing to say to someone with a devastating disease, but honest conversation and true statements are better than fluffy words that are best suited for use as a slogan. It's okay to let the patient know you don't know what to say. It's okay to let them know you are afraid of offending them or making them feel sad with your words or your personal fear of what they are going through. And it's okay to just sit with them, cry with them, listen to them vent, or just share space.

Some of my most comforting times were when people just shared space with me. Every time I was hospitalized, my dear friend Michelle would bring all her "gadgets"—cell phone, laptop, etc.—and work from my hospital room. Sometimes staying an hour or more, often not speaking but just sitting with me and working on her laptop, she shared space and her love.

Tip 1: A good way to get involved is to find out when a patient is going to an appointment or having treatment and then be there for them. I do that with my cancer friends, and they are always genuinely happy to see me, even if I am only there to share a hug. It is surprising how a five-minute visit can carry a patient through an otherwise long, lonely day.

Tip 2: Setting up a meal delivery chain through mutual friends is a great way to be present and available to the patient and their family.

Tip 3: Checking to make sure the patient has adequate transportation to and from appointments is very useful because, most times, we patients either do not feel up to driving or are unable to drive after receiving treatment.

Tip 4: It is also helpful to have someone clean the house, even if that only means the bathroom and the kitchen. My husband did his best to do it all: work, cook, take care of me, clean. But, oh, what

I would have given for a hand in this area, as I felt a lot of guilt by not being able to keep up my own house for a year.

Tip 5: Leading on from the previous tip, another way to provide support is to keep the patient's caregiver in mind. That person has the weight of the world on their shoulders with all the added responsibilities. And don't think the patient doesn't realize this, which in turn adds unhealthy stress to the situation. The sense of guilt that comes with this can at times be overwhelming to the patient. Consider taking the caregiver out for a much-needed cup of coffee or meal, or perhaps sit with the patient so the caregiver can go for a solo walk or on an outing with friends. If the caregiver is running on empty, everyone feels it, so being present and available to the caregiver is a huge help to the patient.

Whatever you do, we do love you for trying: anything is better than nothing. It is on the patient to educate friends and family as much as it is on the non-patient to be sensitive to the irritating little sayings that seem so harmless. Bottom line: most patients would prefer a well-meaning gesture, such as a meal or a visit, to an empty cliché that is better left on a T-shirt or a charity wristband.

PART TWO
Surviving Treatment

The pain, emotional wreckage, debilitation, and the struggle to keep a grip on and maintain mental health.

THE PATIENT

We Are All Here to Teach and to Learn

*The cancer journey can reveal the best of human
nature and bring out the best in you.*

MY HUSBAND'S FAVORITE LINE IS, "There are no accidents." I believe he is
correct. Throughout my journey, I have met some of the most amazing
people, whom I call angels. Apparently, I am not alone in this experience, and I have heard a considerable number of stories about angels
who have been put in front of patients going through their journey.

I met a couple in their eighties who were flying to Houston,
Texas, from Arizona to volunteer at the cancer hospital that saved
the wife's life. I heard stories of volunteers who donate their time in
honor of a loved one. I have loved on dogs brought into the hospital
for comfort during treatment. I have been serenaded by pianists and
singers while receiving infusions and eaten homemade cookies while

in the waiting room. I have had strangers offer to donate blood and bone marrow on my behalf and to puppy-sit while I was in treatment (I am still not sure how that woman actually knew I had a dog).

Angels do such things, selflessly giving of their time, talent, and energy so that patients like me have a little sunshine during our gray days.

The night nurse during my first in-patient chemotherapy stay (I was hospitalized for five days during every round of chemotherapy) did what she called a "touch prayer." She told me to focus on God. She then, ever so lightly, placed her hands on my feet, then my ankles, and so on up my body. She never said another word just kept lightly placing her hands on my body. I had no idea what she meant by "focus on God," so with my eyes closed and mimicking her silence, I recited in my head over and over, "Thank you, God. Please take away my sickness. Please take away my pain." The power of that angel worked that night.

Voices on Earthly Angels

ONE OF KATE'S ANGELS WAS a technician who operated a machine during her treatment. This woman, whom Kate would see twice a week, became a safe haven for Kate's emotional and spiritual needs. "I honestly don't know that I would have survived the cancer and treatment without her," Kate told me.

Anastasia received her best blessing the day she was diagnosed. She tells the story of walking out of the doctor's office after receiving her diagnosis, walking into the waiting room to where her son was sitting, and bawling her eyes out. A stranger got up and comforted Anastasia, telling her, "Go home, cry yourself dehydrated, scream, and do whatever you need to do. Then tomorrow, get up and fight!"

What may be thought of as a little thing by your angels can have the biggest impact: meal delivery, childcare pick-up or drop-off, or putting your name on a prayer roll. These gifts, these little acts of kindness and love, while seemingly small and perhaps thought of as insignificant for the doer, are huge and perhaps lifesaving, like blood and platelet donations, to the receiver.

I initially commuted 1,800 miles one way for my treatment in Houston, Texas. I was given the name of a group of people fittingly called "Ground Angels" who, on a strictly volunteer basis, would pick up patients flying in for treatment. They would drive the patient into the city, get them settled, and then shuttle them back to the airport when they were done. People from this network assisted me in my travels for eight months. Not only saving me hundreds of dollars, but offering me their time, companionship, and comfort as I traveled alone into the scary unknown of my early treatments. (I traveled alone nearly every time because my husband and I could not afford the cost of two flights or for him to take time off work to come with me.)

Cody was a young man of about twenty and the brother of my son's friend. Cody worked in food services in the hospital where I would have my week long stays for my chemo treatment. At least once during each stay, he never failed to put a note on my food tray that read, "Hi Lynda, from Cody," or the tray delivery person would say, "Cody said to tell you, 'Hi.'" My tears of gratitude flowed every time.

Some angels even come in the form of big corporations. I flew Southwest Airlines on nearly all my trips to Houston, sometimes as often as once per week, and had exceptional customer care from them. I was never charged for a change in my flight or a missed flight due to my treatment or from being sick. And all my special need requests (sometimes I needed physical assistance) were met with complete and utter kindness and compassion. They even offered two vouchers per year to fly free during my treatment—one for me and one for my caregiver. And, most importantly, Jody, who took care of all my travel arrangements, would always hang up from speaking with a Southwest employee with tears in his eyes from hearing that person say he or she would keep us in their thoughts and prayers.

But not all angels come in the form of humans; they also appear as our pets. Tucker "Bug," my long-haired miniature dachshund, was an amazing comfort during my worst times. He would lay his little warm body on my lap and not move for hours, just sitting there for me to feel his tiny heart beat as I pet him. He was a true angel in some of my darkest hours. I am not alone with this experience: nearly everyone who had a pet during their treatment has a similar story.

Thank you to all our angels—furry, corporate, and human.

It's My Cancer and I'll Cry If I Want To

Some fears never go away, but it helps to express them and accept help to deal with them.

WE ALL WANT TO BE positive. We all try to be positive. But sometimes, we just can't, and that should be okay. For some reason, however, it isn't. I am not sure why when a person is diagnosed with a debilitating and life-altering or life-ending illness, the world automatically assumes being positive is going to cure everyone's woes.

Positivity is a great state to live in. It is healthy, reduces stress and anxiety, and generally makes a person much easier to be around, but it is not always realistic. There are times when self-pity, anger, sadness, and fear simply take over. And there are times when we just need a good cry, a good scream, or a good pity party. Please let us have it.

On the drive home from a most exasperating oncology appointment, Jody and I counted to three then screamed at the top of our lungs, twice. It felt so good to release the pent up emotions that it brought a wonderful bout of much-needed laughter to both of us, which was much healthier than faking positivity when we both really wanted to, well, scream.

Voices on Emotional and Mental Health

IT'S OKAY TO BE MAD. Cancer is not fair, and no one should be expected to go through it without having moments of doubt, terror, and anger. Being diagnosed with cancer is somewhat similar to losing a loved one. We go through all the same steps of the grieving process—denial, anger, bargaining, depression, and acceptance. We will remain in one step longer than others, breeze through other steps, and keep returning to certain steps. It is a *process*: we need to go through it, and you need to allow it.

Joni (not my cousin), who has NHL, struggles with anxiety

and depression related to her disease. Her significant other does not understand her emotions and feelings and tells her she should just be happy that she is alive. Joni is very happy to be alive but hates treatment and misses her old self, all of which cause her anxiety and depression. The inability to be open about these issues closes her off from her partner because she feels her emotions are not being validated.

Grace, a two-time breast cancer survivor, fell hard into denial during her second round with cancer. It seemed unfathomable to her that she would have to start from scratch and go through her battle again.

After fourteen months in remission from her lymphoma, Kim found herself still struggling and said, "I feel like I've almost bounced back to me, almost. I have weary joints and a little neuropathy but, by and large, I'm me. But in the back of my mind it's there; I can't shake it, and I'm on edge. Every day, I go through the motions and function at a high level. I do what I need to do—work, family, friends ... but I just don't feel like me. I feel like I'm half there, listening, feeling, but not really. Inside I'm irritated by everything and everyone, and I'm waiting but not sure what for. I constantly tell myself I should be grateful—and I am, I really am—but the last couple of months, I've been struggling mentally."

Interesting to note, I have heard from many non-patients, especially caregivers, that they get stuck in their own world of grief and "bargaining process" regarding their loved one's diagnosis. The bargaining stage of grief may occur prior to loss as well as after loss, as an attempt to negotiate pain away. My mother still struggles with the bargaining process two years after my diagnosis. She has said to me previously, "Was there something you could have done differently?" The implied question was clear: "Was there something you could have done to not get cancer?" While she did not intentionally say this to be hurtful, it was paralyzing.

We are a culture of "It's all good" and "No worries," but that is surface nonsense when it comes to fighting for your life; it is not always *all good* and we do worry, even if we say we don't.

It may come as a surprise to learn that, at times, it can be too much to handle when a supporter is filled with unrealistic ideas of rainbows and unicorns regarding our diagnosis, prognosis, or treatment. This is a crappy fight, and we are sick and we are tired, and sometimes your living in la-la land is more than we can take. We want to be positive, and we appreciate you as our cheerleader, but we also need realism. We, better than anyone, understand our bodies, our pain, our ill feelings, our crazy thoughts, our fear, and our grief. And we, better than anyone, understand our prognosis, which for some is terminal.

It is human nature to try to cheer up someone who is in despair, but telling them to "be strong" is not necessarily helpful, and it really doesn't work anyway. People don't want advice on how they should feel ("Look on the bright side") or how to be fixed ("Things will be better tomorrow"); they often just want to be heard.

There is a fine line between positive and unrealistic. Acknowledging a person's pain or bad day, instead of trying to move them past it, is the most helpful way to go. It is not your job to fix me or whatever is wrong with my mental state. It is best to simply say, "I'm sorry you are going through this. Would you like to talk about it?"

Find Others with the Same Diagnosis

Being afraid is one thing. Being alone and afraid is far worse.
Find others who understand your fears and problems.

EARLY IN MY JOURNEY, I found that nothing was off-limits when talking with another cancer patient. It was as if the hospital wristbands worn by patients created an instant bond between us.

I remember the first time I met someone in person who had my exact type of cancer. Having a type of cancer seen predominantly in men, it was no surprise this person was a man with the same diagnosis. Bob became a beacon of hope to me, someone who showed me that I was no longer alone in my fight.

I first met Bob at MD Anderson Cancer Center in Houston, Texas, while we were both doing a clinical drug trial. Bob had flown in from Michigan, and I had come in from Idaho. He was chatting in the lobby with his wife and Jody, while I was getting my labs (blood) drawn. When I came out into the waiting room, Jody introduced me to Bob, saying, "He has mantle cell lymphoma."

I reached out, touched Bob's arm, and choked on my happy tears. "Oh my gosh, I'm not alone." Bob, who was nearly 65 at the time, hugged me to let me know he was real and he was there for me. I still share a wonderful connection with Bob, and we keep track of each other and our health status. He was a testament to the fact that I was not isolated on my own cancer island. Unfortunately, Bob, who started the same month in the clinical trial with me in Houston, has relapsed, twenty-four months after his remission.

I am not alone in my quest to find another inhabitant on my personal solitary, sparsely populated island. We all feel the need to connect with others who share our diagnosis, but sometimes those people are difficult to find—especially when your cancer is rare.

Anastasia, who has fought chronic myelogenous leukemia (CML) for the past several years, had never actually met anyone with her disease. She hails from a postage-stamp-sized town in Mississippi, and her only connection with other CML patients has been online. I was fortunate enough to witness her meet Jay, who has also had CML for several years. In a moment of déjà-vu, I watched as Anastasia reached out, touched Jay's arm, and with tears of joy said, "Oh my God, I am not alone."

The importance of fellowship, companionship, and camaraderie is real to every human being. We all want to fit in, to be a part of a group, and not be an outsider. It is no different in the world of fighting cancer.

At the beginning of my journey, my husband would become almost embarrassed by my brash way of accosting other cancer patients. I would walk right up to a stranger in a waiting room and say, "Hello, my name is Lynda. I have mantle cell lymphoma. What kind of cancer do you have?" And Jody would smile, almost apologetically at his seemingly crazy wife, and shrink away just a bit.

Surprisingly though, I have yet to speak with a fellow patient who didn't want to share something. Even the grumpiest of old men who protested to everyone about everything still wanted to share something.

My husband, my children, and my friends all want to understand what I am going through, and I appreciate their efforts. But unless they have had a cancer diagnosis, they will never fully grasp what it is like. Other cancer fighters know and feel and understand the same things I do; they *get it*. Cancer patients are, therefore, immediately bonded with one another.

Nikko, who battled breast cancer and then leukemia, is a reserved observer of others and felt that no one else had her same thoughts and feelings about cancer. She said that once she learned others shared her fear, hope, and happiness regarding their cancer, she felt validated, as if she were no longer the only one with those feelings. She felt less alone.

What We Worry About

WHAT ARE SOME OF THESE thoughts and feelings?

We think about our death (how can we not?), we think about our life, and our families.

We worry about every scan and the time in between.

We dread the next needle prick and pill to swallow.

We are humiliated by the constant diarrhea. We wish the nausea and vomiting would subside and long for the good old days when we had hair, nice skin, and a healthy weight.

With every lump or bruise, we obsess about whether the cancer is back. We worry about what kind of attack we are having, heart or panic. We feel like we live in a constant hypochondriac state: is it just a cough or am I sick again?

We cry for our children and our loved ones. We fixate on whether our spouse can handle life if we are no longer here. We worry about who will take care of our fur babies.

We wonder what the world will look like when we are gone and if we will be thought of and how.

We panic over our finances.

We wonder if we will ever have a normal sex life again. Some grieve, knowing they will never have a child because they have become sterile from the drugs or surgery.

We wonder if we will be alone, will anyone be there for us, will we find and keep love.

We think about how we may want to end our suffering and what spiritual ramifications that could bring.

We hate the pity when people look at our bald head.

We understand the confusion of others when we say we just don't "feel right."

We feel awkward in a room full of healthy people.

We swallow bitterness when we hear someone complain about a slight sniffle or stubbed toe: we only wish we had it so good.

We know we will never be normal again.

These overwhelming, complex, and sometimes irrational thoughts and feelings will always cause us to feel different from you.

THE NON-PATIENT

When a Physician is Touched by Cancer

The cancer shift perspective through the eyes of those in the healthcare community.

I CANNOT SAY ENOUGH GOOD things about the professional teams of people who assisted me during and after my illness. Healthcare providers are a special kind of people. They hold our hands when we are scared, they stay an extra minute to listen to a story when we are lonely, and they administer lifesaving techniques as a matter of course. And they do it all with a smile. They are amazing individuals.

But what does it look like when *they* or someone they love gets the diagnosis?

My local oncologist is an amazingly tender man who is not afraid to profess his feelings of concern, care, and faith. He would always speak gently to me, touch my arm softly in comfort, and even suggest that I pray to get through my treatment. He is a kind soul, and I hold him in the highest regard. He recommended that my initial treatment should be not be in his care but with a doctor who was a specialist in my specific type of cancer, and in doing so, he likely added time to my life.

Unfortunately, regardless of how kind, how educated or faithful a person, these people are no more immune from the long reach of cancer. My doctor's mother was diagnosed with brain cancer, and although all measures were tried, she succumbed to a complication during one of her procedures. The man I admired so much, who was so well respected in his oncology field and who I was leaning on with my life, watched his mother lose her war with cancer.

It was difficult to see his pain on my visits with him after this. But with his mother's passing, I noticed a shift in him: he became even more than a doctor. He seemed to understand in a much deeper and emotional way when I talked about my symptoms, my fears, my joys. The look in his eyes changed, and I could see that he "got it" on a level beyond doctor to patient. Now he understands on a personal level.

The social worker I see told me a story about my doctor. She said that she ran into him after his mother had passed and told him that she was sorry for his loss. In his usual genuine fashion, he stopped and said poignantly, "Is your mother still alive?" The social worker told him that her mother was still alive, and the doctor said, "You are quite fortunate," and then took the time to speak with her about how she needed to remember to hold her mother close.

I was fortunate to meet Kate, a nurse who survived her breast cancer. She was my caregiver during a particularly slow evening at the hospital, and she shared her story with me. I am unsure if that was because we were both cancer patients or because we were both mothers of three children, but we hit it off and formed a very quick bond. It was a true testament to the type of person a nurse can be.

Kate was in her mid-thirties and thirty-three weeks pregnant with triplets when she received her diagnosis of breast cancer. A devout woman, she felt God would take care of her and the babies long enough to let her deliver prior to treatment for her cancer. She delivered the babies, who were as healthy as triplets could be, and nearly immediately had one of her breasts surgically removed. Her doctor allowed her to keep the other breast so she could nurse her three babies for the first two months of their lives. After the two months was up, Kate returned to the hospital to have her second breast removed.

After her surgeries and chemotherapy, Kate decided to rededicate her life by going back to school and becoming a nurse. She epitomizes the reason people become caregivers: to help others and to give back.

As my chemotherapy required five days' hospitalization each round, I got to know the staff on the cancer floor well. They were all such amazing people—so dutiful, attentive, and full of life; and most of them were so young! I was surprised when I first walked onto the floor at 4 South that nearly everyone there was a millennial. They were all bubbly and fresh, full of vim and vigor, and ready to take on the world. Brea was one of my favorites of those millennials. She had been a nurse for a few years and loved her job on the oncology floor. She had long blonde hair that she always kept pulled back in a youthful ponytail, and she had an infectious personality I could not help but be drawn to.

I would see Brea numerous times during the many weeks I spent on 4 South, and there was never a time she didn't dole out a hug, an enormous smile, and a kind word.

Once I finished treatment, it would be several months before I ran into Brea again on the floor. This time, instead of a long blonde ponytail, she had a beautiful bald head. I asked her, "Is this new look in support of someone or is there something I don't know about?" I knew the answer before she spoke.

Without knowing it was Brea, I had seen her go into the bathroom one day from where I sat for my infusion, and I had heard her vomiting. I watched her go in several times during my stay, assuming it was a patient choosing to use the bathroom in the hall rather than in their room. Unbeknown to me at the time, that person was Brea, running into the bathroom to vomit between caring for her cancer patients. She was obviously now a cancer patient herself. I was in awe.

Voice of a Caregiver with Cancer

WITH BREA'S PERMISSION, I AM sharing something she wrote, as I think it is not only beautiful but necessary to understand how it feels when someone we rely on to take care of us is dealt the same hand as ours:

> *Throughout this journey, I am often asked what it is like to be an oncology nurse while also being a cancer patient. The answer is quite simple, really: it is sacred.*
>
> *Today, I am a cancer patient. I am getting treatment and pecking away at my keyboard as we speak, locking eyes and exchanging waves with the nurses as they scurry by. I*

am but one of many hairless heads sitting in a chair that
is not all that comfy, in a room that is just a little too cold.
Just like every other patient in here, I, too, cringe at the chill
that's accompanied by the blood pressure cuff that is still wet
from a sanitizer cloth. I, too, hold my breath as the needle is
plunged into the port in my chest. I, too, know the dizzying
effect that takes place in my body when all the pre-medications
swirl together in opposition. I, too, know the toxic feeling that
swells in my throat when the chemotherapy starts dripping,
a little unnerved by the fact the nurse has to put on a practi-
cal hazmat suit just to administer it. I also crane my neck to
watch the noxious fluid fall methodically, shutting my eyes for
just a second to pray it is doing its job. I am also frustrated by
the sticky wheel on my IV pump, making it feel as if I'm drag-
ging a stubborn child to the bathroom. I catch a gaze from
another human with a kind face and tired eyes; we exchange
warm smiles and a nod of encouragement.

Tomorrow, I will be your oncology nurse. I will rest,
hydrate, and eat as I am supposed to today so I have the
energy to care for you in the fullest. I will fill my soul with
sunshine and the love of my friends and family, so I may be an
outlet for your frustrations. I will pray and burn through all
of the worries on my mind tonight so I can listen to you with
my undivided, sincerest attention. Hearing all about your
family camping trip, your son's soccer game last weekend, and
your plans for your summer break from high school is something I cherish. If I need to, I will smile, and I will cry for
myself tonight so I can do the same for you tomorrow. I will
be sure to remind the people supporting me through this how
grateful I am for them today so that I may hold your hand

and support you. If you are ready, I will take on the honor of shaving your head; we will sit on your bed and giggle as we trial a headscarf fashion show.

I will let my personal experience make me more cognizant and intentional in how we interact tomorrow, but I will not let my diagnosis take my focus off you. Your eyes will dance back and forth from the photo on my badge of the long-haired blonde to my now hairless head. Your natural curiosity will prompt you to ask, and I will be honest with you. You will try and compare our battles; I won't let you.

I will never, ever understand what you are going through ... not fully. As a wise soul once told me, as cancer patients we are all in different lanes. We may be on the same freeway headed to the same destination, but right now I am in the carpool lane on cruise control with a car full of people that love me. You may be in the same lane with a little bump in the road; you may be stopped on the shoulder with a flat tire, out of gas, and no one in sight.

But let me tell you something: if my battle with cancer helps me to understand any part of what you are going through a little bit better, it is worth it. It is sacred. You have humbled me. You have broken and rebuilt me completely, just in a day's work. You are my respite, even if our day together is long and taxing. You fill me. I am who I am because of you, and I am grateful for you.

Today, I am a cancer patient so that I can be your nurse tomorrow.

Dark Thoughts Unspoken

Some thoughts are so fearful or negative or humiliating
they may seem best unshared because they might be
misunderstood by someone without a cancer diagnosis—but
they are human nature and they need to be expressed.

I BELIEVE IT IS SAFE to say that those of us struggling with a chronic illness reach a point in our journey where we start to keep both the little and the big stuff to ourselves. We may tell you in a clinical, matter-of-fact way about our upcoming procedures, our medications, our aches and pains, but we keep our inner feelings out of it. We keep the tough stuff locked behind closed doors—the stuff that would make our family weep and our friends run away. In my world, I call these "thoughts unspoken." My husband calls this me "being in my head."

These *thoughts* have come from dozens of people with whom I have talked:

"I was scared but felt I couldn't share that with many."

"What happens to those deep, dark thoughts? Those 'what ifs' that are not so far from the surface every moment of the day? I even wake up thinking about 'it.'"

"It's always on my mind. I keep thinking I am going to wake up from this. I think, 'Can I beat this?' 'How much has it spread?' 'Will I see my daughters grow up and get married?'"

"I always try to stay positive, but right now I just want to scream and cry a little. I have an amazing support system here, but sometimes I feel like I can't cry or be mad because they think I'm not being positive."

"Some days I cry more than others, and other days I am totally fine and at peace with what is happening."

"My mind is spinning."

"I am tired of being in pain."

"I am seeing a psychologist."

"I cried out to God for help!"

"I am angry at cancer."

"I am angry that everyone else gets to have a normal life."

"I am frustrated by 'chemo brain,' the memory loss, and the fog."

"I wonder, would others be able to smile if they were in my place? Would they say they are fine when they are screaming to quit and [want to] run away?"

"I feel so much pressure on myself to be able to be the mom, wife, employee that I used to be."

"Do you think we will ever get to the point where the thoughts of it returning do not consume us?"

"I lack motivation now; I just want to stay in my house."

"I am overwhelmed when I see that someone on our cancer [support] page relapses or dies, wondering when that will be me."

"Is this really my life?"

"If this gets too bad, I will find a gun."

"Yes, I believe in assisted suicide."

"In my state, we can use medical marijuana to help with the side effects, and I do."

"In my state, we can't use medical marijuana, but I still do."

"I just want a normal sex life, intimacy, physical connection."

"Where are you? I want to ask my friends."

"I didn't want to talk to anyone. I just kept to myself. I self-isolated."

"They [non-patients] don't get it; they never will. There is no way they can really understand what we are going through, and it isn't their fault."

"I don't want to save for the future anymore; I won't be there. I want to spend money and enjoy it now."

"I want to max out every credit card, move to Cancun for the next few years and get drunk on the beach every day."

"The future stresses me out, and I lose perspective."

"Don't waste my time."

For me, the weeks following my diagnosis were a blur. I vacillated between sobbing and hypersensitivity. I spent time cleaning out my closet, rationalizing that I didn't want my family to have to do this after I was dead. I made piles to give away and piles that I would hang onto until my demise. I found and read each letter and note that I had kept over the years, reminiscing with smiles and tears the memories of my past. I looked through an old box that held pictures and mementos of my boys through their growing-up years; all the hand-crafted macaroni necklaces and Mother's Day cards professing I was the best mom in the world. This would land me in a heap on my closet floor in the midst of the photos and cards, weeping at the thought of never seeing my children again and whispering, "Oh my God, I am going to die."

I met with an attorney and drafted up a will, a power of attorney and healthcare directive. I reached out to a funeral home to get my affairs in order, choosing cremation as my end on this earth. It seemed wasteful to spend money on a casket if my body was withered and unrecognizable from the war it would likely wage at the end. I kept these events and excursions to myself, never sharing with anyone.

Conversations with my husband became sharp and to the point. I looked at life as if it was ending immediately for me, and I needed to make sure I took full advantage of the moments I had.

I remember one breakfast when I just blurted out, "I want you to get remarried after I die."

"What?" Jody said, nearly choking on his eggs.

"I don't want you to be alone. You will still be young, and I want you to be happy." Then, because I thought it would be helpful and make him more comfortable if I approved of his future spouse, I told him, "I will help you pick out your next wife if you'd like." That was the end of that conversation. It was really bad on all kinds of levels, and Jody was having no part of my hysteria.

My brain moved at what felt like lightning speed after my diagnosis. I had a great sense of urgency to move forward with my life quickly, while still taking the time to enjoy everything along the way.

I had some very irrational thoughts as I tried to rationalize my diagnosis. There was a time when I actually wished I had breast cancer, as I thought it was an *easy* cancer. I was bitter because I didn't have the pink cancer. Everything I had heard was that breast cancer was nearly always curable. Ads all over television and the internet promote "pink in support of breast cancer." There are fun runs and charity events, and legislation on insurance specifically regarding breast cancer. There are clinical trials and monies to be given to those needing tests and treatment, and there are shirts with catchy sayings, such as, "Save the Ta-Tas," and "Race for the Cure." No other cancer has near as much publicity, camaraderie, or money being raised and donated as breast cancer. I was jealous and envious. I wanted the type of cancer that people would race for. I wanted to have a recognized cancer support color. Lime green, my cancer support color, is flashy but it will never be pink. I wanted to be able to say, "Yes," when people looked at me as a female with cancer and nearly always said matter-of-factly, "Oh, breast cancer?"

Not only did I not have breast cancer, I had an incurable,

male-dominated blood cancer. Ugh. I actually went so far as to purposefully not wear pink in the beginning so my bald head would not be automatically associated as me having breast cancer. I felt distant and disconnected from these *pink* women. I missed out on the camaraderie I saw when they would talk amongst themselves about their disease, their treatment, and their cancer-specific issues. I felt like the outcast in junior high, trying but not fitting into the in-crowd, not having the "cool kid's cancer."

And it is with shame that I admit I thought it would have been so much easier to have breast cancer. I thought a breast could be removed but blood could not—so it must be easier. I learned later that I, like a lot of people, was undereducated and naïve when it came to breast cancer. What bothered me the most about breast cancer had also misinformed me the most: the hype.

I realize that reading that section may be infuriating to some, but I am writing this to be as transparent as possible and let people know what goes on in the heads of patients—the good, the bad, and the unthinkable. For anyone with breast cancer, please accept my sincere apology for my ignorance.

Fortunately, life has a funny way of putting people in front of you just when you need them. And fittingly, just as I needed it, I found myself at a camp for adult cancer survivors surrounded by women who had breast cancer. Through those women, I was able to cleanse my soul of my horrible thoughts, tell them how much I resented not being able to play in the sandbox with them, and then get educated to the nth degree on what breast cancer really looked like: the pain, the humiliation, the suffering, the loss of femininity, the insecurities.

I also learned things the internet and commercials don't tell you, including the separation of the patients with stage 4. Their support color once their cancer metastasizes is no longer pink. It is white.

Those patients with stage 4 breast cancer I spoke with felt as if they were kicked out of the so-called cool kids' cancer club.

Statistics show that in the United States, someone dies from breast cancer every 14 minutes and that metastatic breast cancer is the only breast cancer that is a killer. Yet only 2 to 5 percent of funds raised for breast cancer research are spent on studies of metastasis.[3] Furthermore, all the charity walks and buying of pink merchandise is not working: the number of deaths from breast cancer has not significantly decreased in over forty years.

I had one stage 4 breast cancer patient tell me, "The doctors don't do anything for us; they feel there is nothing they can do." She went on to tell me she will continue taking her oral chemo pills until the day she dies or until she decides she is done—these are the only options she has been given.

Suffice it to say, a lot of tears were shed, a lot of ah-ha moments were had by me, and incredible new bonds, built on raw and open communication, were formed during those days I spent learning about breast cancer. I can say now with all honesty, I would never wish to have "their kind of cancer" any more than my own. Such thinking is crazy.

The crazy thoughts unspoken don't end when we hear the words "complete remission" (CR), "no evidence of disease" (NED) or "no evidence of active disease" (NEAD). I continued internalizing my fear even after I showed no signs of active disease, withdrawing from everyone but keeping a façade of happiness with a smile on my face, a laugh in my voice, and a superficiality in my conversation. Yes, I had terminal cancer. Yes, my prognosis was still a few short years. Yes, I was scared. And yes, at times I avoided it all together.

I put my energy into helping my friends and family feel comfortable with the realities of my cancer, as doing so kept me from getting too overwhelmed with my own fear of my mortality. I was going to die, much sooner than I ever anticipated.

When It's Time to Say Goodbye

THE REALITY IS THAT NOT everyone who is diagnosed with cancer will survive. The variables as to who will make it through and who will not are as vast as the number of stars in the sky. The truth is there will be many of you reading this who will face the most difficult decisions and times of your life while watching your loved one battle for the last few days of their life. The key is remembering that this is *their life*, not yours. You must recognize when your loved one can no longer fight. When the treatments and the side effects are wearing out their body and their spirit to the extent that they are doing more damage than good.

We all want our loved ones with us forever, and we patients don't want to die—but that is not realistic, and it is not for those without cancer to choose for the patient when enough is enough. If your loved one is done fighting, respect that. Acknowledge your feelings with him or her, but if you are honest, most of those feelings of letting them go will simply be fear, "How do I live my life without you?" and "What if this one more treatment could be the cure?" You will live without them; you will be in an altered state, but you will live. As for that additional treatment, if the patient is not physically or mentally capable of accepting it, it won't work anyway.

As the patient, we know how it feels to treat, to be tested, to wait for results. We are familiar with the side effects of pain, nausea, diarrhea, fatigue, memory loss, and word-searching problems. We know we are not our old selves, and we also know no matter how hard we try, we will never be our old selves again. And we know when we cannot take any more.

We know when it is time to let go. Please, let us go with dignity and without guilt for wanting to rest.

Happy Thoughts Unspoken

Good can come from thinking about and facing your own death. It's about understanding life.

AS HORRENDOUS AND AWFUL AS cancer sounds, it isn't all bad. There is clarity to everything I see. I liken it to a newborn kitten whose eyes have just opened. My eyes have been opened like never before.

The haze of the everyday mundane fades away and is replaced by brighter, crisper colors and sharper images. Things just *feel* better in an introspective way; as if my personal aura is healthier, purer, more open and inviting and accepting of things and people in a more gracious way.

An interesting example is that I now have a "thing" for squirrels. I always thought they were cute, but now I actually pay attention to them. I enjoy watching them scurry around and chase after each other, and I chuckle when I find a peanut planted in my garden and hope the little guy who stole my flower bulb got a good meal out of it. My previous self would have chased the little beggar off with a broom and some expletives.

Things don't seem to bother me like they once did, and I am far more tolerant, almost to a fault. One of my common phrases of late is, "I don't care." My meaning is neither sarcastic nor said out of irritation. It is honest; I simply don't care much about anything when it comes to strife or conflict. I would rather capitulate than argue, even when I know I am right.

There are no more "discussions" about what to eat for dinner, which toothpaste my husband should have bought, or why my kids are late for dinner. I don't care about those things and am just happy now to have a full belly, clean teeth, and see my children when they drop in, late or not.

Prior to my diagnosis, I was a very happy person and led a good, full life with little or no complaints. I feel even happier now and find myself smiling even more. My smile is not only outward now but inward, and my self-talk is positive, kind, and forgiving of others as well as of myself.

I am grateful for everything and every day, and that is no longer just words I feed myself from Post-it notes stuck to my mirror as *positive affirmations*. This behavior has now become second nature, and it appeared only after being diagnosed and going through terrific suffering and struggles. In my world today, I am often surprised when I wake up in the morning, saying to myself, "Wow, I got to wake up again!" Life truly is a gift, and I am so thankful to have it.

When I was terribly sick, I learned that time was not necessarily my friend. I was bound to it like a slave. It commanded when I woke up and set the times when I would eat. It told me when to use the bathroom and when to go to work; it ran my life. During my sickest days, I learned to sleep when I was tired, wake when I was done sleeping, eat when I was hungry, and work when I was able.

After I began to recover from those sick days, I remained vigilant about not running my life by time. I still don't have a clock by my bedside. I eat when I am hungry, even if that means lunch at 10:00 a.m. or dinner at 10:00 p.m. I work when I feel capable, and I don't push it when my energy is running thin. I have found balance, and with that came peace and contentment that no self-help book has ever been able to give me.

I no longer worry about the grass on the other side of the fence, as my grass looks just fine, dandelions and all. My hope for those who have not found this perspective is that they are given the opportunity one day to see life through an uncluttered lens where hope is abundant and life is *felt* as a gift.

Voices on Good Thoughts

I AM NOT ALONE IN this newfound perspective of clarity following extreme suffering. My little chemo-brain notebook of "reminders" holds the following statements from others that I found worthy of penning.

"My perspective now that I am in remission is that life is uncomplicated, if you let it be."

"I am a better version of me because of the battle I fight."

"I have a feeling of peace and stillness."

"I stopped focusing on the noise of the world."

"Things just seem better now."

"I don't take *anything* for granted."

"My heart is full of gratitude for life."

"Cancer is a scurrilous menace and can repeatedly lay you flat. But by the grace of God, I keep popping up again."

"Cancer has gotten my attention, and now I am much more in tune with my body."

"I celebrate what's really important; I am alive this day."

"I want to make an impact."

"I realize now people are more important than getting things done."

"*Aut viam inveniam aut faciam.*" (I will either find a way or make one.)—Hannibal, 247–182 B.C.), as quoted by a cancer patient.

PART THREE

Forward into the New Normal

Once you have faced what could kill you, there's no going back.

THE PATIENT

What Does My New Normal Look Like?

The definition of "normal" changes when you have cancer. Appearances can be deceiving.

A YOUNG FRIEND OF MINE, Jenna, commented: "There is a constant feeling of need to explain. I have a handicap placard, and you should see the looks I get."

Jenna has a bone disease where her body literally fuses itself together. She is only twenty-four years old, looks completely healthy, and is full of life, like any other woman her age. However, she suffers with immense pain and physical issues because of her unseen illness. She is in constant pain and requires regular infusions and medications similar to those taken by cancer patients.

Regarding her placard, Jenna continued: "When I get out of the car, I look totally fine. I put my handicap placard in the window, and

I feel like I need to tell everyone who's looking what is wrong with me, like I need to justify why, at my age, looking perfectly normal, I need a handicap spot. I tend to hang my head a bit, almost ashamed, whenever I notice someone watching me use my placard."

I completely understand this feeling, as I too have a handicap placard now, and I too hang my head a bit when I use it. In my situation, pain can come on quickly and change my ability to walk in a matter of hours. Interestingly, when I need my cane to assist me in walking, people passing by generally look at me with pity mixed with a smile, which tells me how brave they think I am. There is no "shame on you" look when I use my placard in these situations. But when I hang the placard and walk away from my car without the cane, the looks tend to be more an indignant scoff. Do I need to show them that I carry a cane in my bag *just in case*?

"Normal"—What We Were Before Cancer

WHY IS IT THAT THOSE of us who have been diagnosed say we are not normal or that we will never be normal again? There are two distinctions to our change: the obvious external physical changes and the unseen internal changes.

The scars from surgeries, signs of radiation treatments, physical anomalies in the way we walk, talk, or behave, or loss of body parts are the obvious outward signs of the changes. The not-so-obvious change is the way we *feel*, *think*, and *see* things differently than before we began fighting for our lives.

My type of cancer does not warrant radiation or surgical intervention. I cannot speak to those treatments with any authority and can only ask others what it is like to endure those things.

KC has stage 4 sinus cancer and required daily radiation for weeks. Prior to this, he had to have all metal fillings removed from his teeth (which in some cases could mean the removal of the tooth). He was then fitted with a metal plate that fit perfectly to his mouth and down his throat (he had to learn to swallow and tolerate the metal blocker without gagging or moving at any time during the procedures). This metal plate was to protect his tongue, throat, and opposite side of his face from the proton radiation beam. A mesh-like mask that looked like something a knight would wear was placed over his face. As a result of his treatments, KC lost all sense of taste and smell and is plagued with chronic seizures. But he *looks* normal.

Susan told me she felt "gender neutral," after she lost her breasts. She said that when her hair was gone (which included eyebrows and lashes) and her breasts had been removed, people would address her generically as, "Hey man," or "dude." She felt like an outcast because of her lack of specific gender identity.

She opted to have her breasts replaced to give her back her feminine identity. Unfortunately, through a complicated treatment course and nearly every issue imaginable, nine surgeries, and the removal of one of her implants, Susan has still not fully reconstructed her damaged body. But to look at her, you would never know she had ever been sick. She is extremely active, and she loves kayaking and running marathons.

Pam, another breast cancer survivor, opted not to have her breasts reconstructed because she felt it was better for her body not to undergo the process of reconstruction. Instead, she took on the challenge of the stares and the questioning looks of a life as a woman with no breasts. "I felt my boobs had served their purpose. And it is so fab with no bra and all that goes with it," Pam told me. She also shared what she calls a fun fact: she cannot be convicted of indecent exposure by going topless as a female because she has no nipples ... I would never have thought about that.

Michael, a testicular cancer survivor, opted in his early twenties to preserve his ability to father children by foregoing chemotherapy. He chose the radical route of having his diseased testicle and lymph nodes removed. Michael now has a prosthetic testicle.

While completely different issues, KC, Susan, Pam, and Michael have a lot in common—sharing feelings of fear, anxiety, and being overwhelmed at times regarding their physical changes. All of them, however, would prefer to talk about what they have been through than pretend it doesn't exist.

Looks Can Be Deceiving

CANCER ALSO TAKES AWAY THINGS that are unseen but which can be just as difficult as physical scars.

I was a dancer. I never competed, nor did I perform, but I loved to dance. I found it therapeutic at a time in my life when I was looking for a healthy outlet. I had always wanted to dance, so one day I answered an ad on Craigslist:

Professional dancer seeks partner. Must be 5'2"–5'4" tall,
weigh no more than 120 pounds, live locally, and be available
after hours. No experience necessary. Will teach for free.

I thought this sounded perfect; my friends thought I would end up dead in a basement somewhere. Fortunately, I was right, and I did learn to dance. My instructor became a lifelong friend who would ultimately teach my husband how to dance as well.

Three to five nights per week, I was out on the dance circuit, laughing with friends, and grooving to anything with a beat. I would ballroom, salsa, swing, and country dance. I wasn't the best dancer, but I had a great time. I was in amazing shape and had more energy than most.

Slowly, however, I was getting tired and winded while dancing, and every few months I felt as if I had the flu. I chalked my symptoms up to overworking, raising kids, or eating the wrong foods. Ultimately, of course, I was diagnosed with cancer, which changed my normal forever.

As I write this, I am currently on maintenance immunotherapy infusions only. I will receive these infusions every other month for two years. These infusions consist of a drug that is an antibody against the specific protein found in persons with my type of cancer. When the antibody binds to that specific protein, it triggers cell death, which will keep my cancer dormant—hopefully. Because this drug is relatively easy for me to handle, I refer to these infusions as "baby chemo," whereas my in-patient chemotherapy is a "nuclear bomb." My grueling days of trial drugs and chemotherapy are behind me for now, and today I look normal. I have hair, eyebrows, and eyelashes. My skin is a normal color, and my weight is back. But I still have not been able to get back out on the dance floor like I once did; I simply do not have the stamina and am plagued by fatigue.

I read an article titled "Post-Cancer Fatigue: The Invisible Wound," written by Kathy LaTour.[4] In this article, LaTour accurately describes how fatigue is an ongoing, dominant issue following cancer treatment, which 75–100 percent of survivors face. This fatigue, which is unique to cancer patients, is referred to as cancer-related fatigue (CRF). According to this article, CRF is defined as "fatigue that is out of the ordinary, not the kind from jet lag or a poor night's sleep or being up with a newborn and not relieved by sleep or rest. This fatigue ranges from lacking enough energy to stand up to never regaining former levels [of stamina]."

Reading this article helped validate my own fatigue issues and was instrumental in helping my husband understand what I mean when I say, "I am just *so* tired."

Chemotherapy does a number on a body and the lasting side effects, while often invisible, are real and daunting. Chemo knocked my balance out of whack, which still sometimes leaves me with difficulties walking straight. I required balance retraining in order to stop bumping into things and listing like a ship ready to capsize.

I also had dramatic, noticeable memory deficits and severe word-searching issues following chemotherapy. I assume these issues are somewhat like those a stroke victim goes through. Mid-sentence, my mind would suddenly go blank as if I had not been just speaking. What I ate for breakfast was forgotten before noon, and I couldn't recall last night's movie or people's names. Words I had used my entire life would roll around inside my head but fail to hit my tongue. I would feel the eternal seconds tick by as I grappled to fill gaps in my sentences with words that should have been easy for me to articulate. As a wannabe wordsmith who has worked in the legal field for thirty years, this was a devastating issue for me, yet one that could not be seen by others. I would be left embarrassed, flabbergasted, concerned, and pissed off.

It is exhausting explaining over and over again that yes, I am doing great and I feel fantastic, but I still cannot do the things I once did. I am not sure if I ever will. It is unbelievably painful to realize and admit to myself and others that I may never put on my dance shoes and really kick up my heels again. I have had to learn that I must stop gauging my abilities by the standard of previous (pre-cancer) me and must instead embrace the present me and my current capacity.

I have pain in my back and neck now, as well as my two middle fingers, right wrist, and left knee. This pain lives with me daily. I have arthritic degeneration, I am told, which is something I never had before all the drugs I was given to help save my life.

I struggle with sudden bouts of dizziness that have left me in a heap on the floor. There is no medical explanation for this, but that is no comfort when the problem is real and my face is on the floor.

My vision is a challenge now, too, and my world is blurry, even with a new prescription.

My ovaries shut down with the first dose of chemo, and in order to stave off the volcanic eruptions of heat from inside my body (hot flashes), I take synthetic hormones. These, of course, can give me breast cancer—just one more concern. And I now require frequent naps in order to get through most days. But to look at me, I *appear* normal.

I have met people who, following chemotherapy treatment, have permanent neuropathy (pain, tingling, and burning sensations) in their fingers and feet. I know people who can no longer work due to the neurotoxicity (damage to the brain, which can affect cognitive skills) caused by the chemotherapy. I have seen a leukemia patient whose legs spontaneously erupted with massive bruising from overexertion (while on vacation, this former performing dancer had simply walked too long for her fragile body; that was her *over-exertion*). I know others who can no longer climb a flight of stairs from the damage their medications have caused their hearts. But they all *look* normal.

Patience is imperative; patience from the patient and for the patient. At times, I see the frustration in my family and friends. They cannot fix me, and they wonder how long this phase is going to last, or they forget why I even have issues. They can see me trying to find words to say or remember stories or stay awake through a movie, but my mind and body still fail me occasionally.

I have had to learn to accept this new me and make peace with sharing space in my body with the vile cells that have so incredibly betrayed me, changed me forever, and still seek to kill me.

Survivor's Guilt

Survivor's guilt is real even among those with cancer. Accept this aspect of human nature and celebrate the successes in your own journey.

ONE OF THE MOST DIFFICULT funerals I ever attended was that of my friend, Ray. He would be the first in my cancer circle to succumb to his disease. His death forced me to seriously face my own mortality for the first time.

I was surprised that I would feel guilt at Ray's passing. I had gone through only a few months of Ray's illness with him and his family. I was an outsider, just beginning her journey, who made a friend in Ray along the way.

After Ray's death I only saw his wife, Diane, twice. We chatted from time to time, and we would send heartfelt texts and well-meaning emails. But we never quite reconnected. For over a year, I was not well enough to leave my house for much more than treatment and doctor's appointments, let alone to meet up with friends. As for Diane, she was a grieving widow learning the daily operations of the farm Ray left behind. She was consumed by her loss and her new role, so she didn't have much available time either. But I always wondered if I were too great a reminder of Ray's illness and death. This thought left me with my first taste of survivor's guilt.

Chris, a NHL patient, had guilt thrust upon him when an acquaintance expressed her anger toward him, "It's not fair that you're still alive and my father isn't." Chris explained that he suddenly felt guilty for living when this young girl's father had lost his cancer battle.

Cecilia didn't feel that she was *sick enough* to be included in the breast cancer sisterhood because she "only needed a partial mastectomy." She actually came to me in tears, telling me she did not require chemotherapy or radiation and felt guilty that she only had, "a little cancer."

Many cancer patients carry guilt, knowing they are thriving when others are not. Our sense of worth can get skewed when the health of a fellow cancer patient friend is declining. We are left wondering why we are having good days, why we are surviving. It is curious that *survivor's guilt* could befall a cancer patient.

"Rodney was like an ox," I was told by his family. "Tougher than most, and there wasn't a thing he couldn't do." Rodney was in his early seventies when I met him, and he also had mantle cell lymphoma. He and I we were initially treated at the same hospital. He was the pillar of health until his diagnosis, and he would succumb to the disease only seventeen months into it, never experiencing the relief of remission. I have outlived "The Ox." I carry some guilt for that, as well as for reaching remission, something Rodney never got. Rodney's sweet wife told me there was no need to feel guilty because we all have a journey. I appreciated the sentiment but still carried the burden of survival.

It is a difficult balance between wanting to celebrate good test results and clear scans and keeping the good news quiet when those around you are failing to thrive. We all want to be healthy and happy, and we all have loved ones who are praying for the miracle that some get and others do not. Surviving can come with a heavy mental price.

Life Is Not About the Things We Have; It's About the Memories We Make

Learn to live in the moment and find joy in small things.

I HAVE LEARNED THAT WHILE many of us are on this journey, we each travel our own path. There are no two individuals who feel the same, think the same, or believe exactly the same. I cannot even begin to imagine what another person feels like through their cancer experience. I can only ask questions and try to relate. However, one thing we do all seem to have in common is the strong desire to make memories while we can.

I heard a story from a friend about a young couple with small children. The husband had been diagnosed with cancer and would not survive. The children, through their wise parents, were taught that life was about memories, not things. At one of the last family outings they had, my friend gave one of the little boys a toy water gun. And while he wanted the water gun, the little boy knew he needed his mother's permission as he was not normally allowed to play with guns of any sort. His mother agreed he could keep the water gun and said to him, "What do you say?" Rather than responding with the typical "thank you," the little boy blessed my friend with a lesson, saying: "Life is not about the things we have; it's about the memories we make."

This heartwarming story made me pause for a moment when I heard it. As a young child, that little boy with the water gun had to learn that memories of his father were all he was going to carry with him into adulthood, that no material item would ever replace his dad or bring him back. He was taught to live in the moment.

How to Live in the Moment

WE OFTEN TALK ABOUT LIVING in the moment, but how do you do that?

Don't multitask while in the presence of others. Put your phone away and take your hands off the keyboard. You cannot give someone the time or the respect they deserve if your phone is lying on the table when you are out with friends or you are typing an email to someone while talking to another. What does your friend feel when you pick up your phone to look at it or continue to click away while they are with you? They conclude that something or someone else is more important.

I put my phone away while out in public now. I have purposefully begun greeting people on the street with, "Hello," or "Good morning." It is almost comical to see the expressions on people's faces as we pass and I actually speak directly to them. Granted, many do not notice me as they pass by with their headphones plugged into their ears or while their heads are down as they wildly exercise their thumbs on their phones. Nonetheless, I made it a new habit, and I enjoy the smiles I do get in return.

Don't waste my time. This little phrase is my motto, post-diagnosis. I have an incredible sense of urgency about my life; I want to experience every sunrise and sunset, watch my dog play, see my children flourish, and capture all of life's wonderful happenings. But I don't have a lot of time to do that, so I have learned to cull the inconsequential goings-on in my days and only give time and attention to the people and things that matter to me, that make me happy, bring me peace, satisfy my needs, and fulfill my life. Everything else, well that's just meaningless fodder that wastes my time.

Do not dwell on the past, and do not focus solely on the future or you will lose what is available right now—the memories of the present. Making those memories will allow your toy water gun to be more special.

Maintaining Momentum

The rest of your life is ahead of you. This is true for all people—no matter how much time you have. And no one really knows how much time they have.

"MY HEART IS FULL OF gratitude for life and embracing the health that was so in jeopardy." Susan wrote these words two years after her bout with breast cancer. For most of us going through this illness, we too look at life as a blessing, a miracle, a gift.

Cancer changes a person forever; there is no going back to the pre-diagnosis life. Some of us must figure out how to accept the scars and the physical differences we now have. We must learn to accept that we may have missing or replacement body parts. And some of us must get used to different colored or curly hair, compliments of chemotherapy. We may now walk and talk differently and must learn to accept this.

My transformation through cancer came from the inside; I feel like I have a visible aura of peace now as I have become what I believe to be a vessel of hope with my new life.

Before I was diagnosed, I was a happy person and, I believe, a genuinely giving person, but I was not always content. In many ways, I felt broken. Previously, I had a lack of certainty regarding who I was, but now I feel like an active participant in my life with my old identity replaced by a life of significance and meaning.

My diagnosis, while devastating, has shaped my present and future, teaching me to lead with love and with a servant's heart. I have been forced to learn to just *be*. And with that stillness came the understanding of reflection to acknowledge, accept, and transform.

Through my pain and suffering, I had clarity of self and people, whom I believe are generally all good. I see the world as a better place and with clearer eyes. I can find rainbows and happiness more easily and have learned to let go of the insignificant and the stressful; I am able to focus on the important.

I am far from perfect, and some parts of me, no matter how hard I try, will never change. I am still quick to react and sharp of tongue, but I am also quick now to accept and acknowledge these deficits and make amends; I have no time to hold on to grudges.

I have learned to set boundaries for my health and my heart. I understand that it is okay to have a voice, even if it isn't popular. I am completing things on my "unfinished list" and feel much joy and accomplishment for it. I have even read the Book of Revelation, and so far, I have not been struck down.

We are all facing a death sentence, but some of us have the fortune of knowing more accurately how much time we have left on this earth. For that, I am the lucky one, and I have chosen to use my knowledge of time to reach out to those who have had an effect on my life. I have been able to say to these people the three most powerful words: "I love you."

I am not sure how long I will feel good, and I do not know exactly when I will relapse or even die, but I do know that while I would not have picked this journey, I would not give up the experience or the new perspectives I have gained. I have become more tolerant, more accepting, more open, and more calm. I no longer need to win all the battles, and I genuinely prefer not to even be involved in any. I do not need your acceptance or approval, and if you don't like me, that's okay too: I will just walk away—no harm, no foul.

My life is far less complicated. I am truer to myself with my feelings, and I express even the ugly stuff with honesty. After all, my feelings are valid, even if they are not popular. Somewhere along this journey, I have even learned to really like myself, including the not so glamorous parts. I have gained both an outward and inward confidence, and it shows. I have become a better version of me through my adversity.

I hope the thoughts and experiences shared by me and my cancer circle have enlightened you to our world and dispelled some of the mysteries of the cancer patient. The fear that comes with this diagnosis can be paralyzing and cause inaction—it can also be overwhelming and cause denial. Both are understandable and acceptable in the short term but need to be overcome. Do nothing to rectify these feelings and you may lose your relationship with your loved one. Do what is necessary to get past the fear so that you can stand with your loved one and face this disease together, and you will find an abundance of growth and love.

Clarity and Perspective

"Thousands of candles can be lit from a single candle, and the life of the candle will not be shortened. Happiness never decreases by being shared." —Buddha

CLARITY AND PERSPECTIVE ARE WHY I would not want to go back to my previous normal.

I find that now the sun shines brighter and things just randomly make me smile. The little things mean so much more and life is just better, happier, and more joyful. I have learned the lessons that in order to understand happiness, one must know sorrow, and in order to understand good health, one must experience physical suffering.

I recently caught myself looking at a cyclist in the driving lane next to me. As I drove by, I smiled because I noticed that the cyclist's arm was very shapely and I thought to myself, "You go, girl!" I was proud of this unknown woman. And while I could not stop to tell her so, I hope somehow my positivity and light shone on her. These little things now make big impacts on me, and I actually look for that woman on the bike when I drive that familiar road. I appreciate her dedication and her physique, and she inspires me with her willingness to ride, rain or shine. I smile every time I am fortunate enough to see her.

When I was first diagnosed, I was told my cancer was very rare and, in my case, it was even rarer because I was a young female. I was also told it was extremely aggressive, with no survivors. I was accepted as a patient by a specialist 1,800 miles away who was world renowned for his work with mantle cell lymphoma. I started a trial drug in the hope of doubling my life expectancy. The drug worked to the extent that it made the cancer dormant, but it wreaked havoc on my joints. The pain was excruciating for eight months. (Please note: I have gone through natural child birth, so I know pain!)

The pain of my trial brought clarity to me in ways that I never want to lose. It allowed me to know what is important in life, and to appreciate the tiniest of things. I would sit, often for hours, without being able to move, just looking out the window. I was unable to watch television—too difficult on my eyes; listen to music— too painful to my head; browse on my iPad—too strenuous to my finger and wrists; or speak—too distracting from the focus it took to manage the pain. Through my pain and my inability to move, my world became small, confined to what I could see through the picture window from where I sat.

When your world is small, devoid of extraneous noise and thought, life becomes clear, focused, and you can see it with a new perspective. You see the value of things beyond yourself, and you are forced to slow down, sometimes being nothing but still. Your eyes begin to open to the ins and outs of everyday life that you once rushed past so as not to be late. There is much peace and personal growth in times of suffering.

As the days passed and my pain continued, I stayed in the same spot on my couch for months, but every day, I felt more of a connection with life as I stared out the window. I often felt I had little more in my world to think about than the squirrels I could see scurrying around.

I learned there is beauty in everything and that peace is most prevalent when we are quiet and still. At times, I thought I might go insane with the pain, but as I could not move, I learned to quiet myself and find my center. I began to see beyond what was outside my window, beyond the squirrels, and began to understand what life meant to me; *my meaning of life.*

I heard a story while at Epic Experience, the camp in Colorado for cancer survivors that I attended, which reminded me of my pain-filled days where I found my peace, my understanding of life, my perspective. It was a story by Robert Fulghum, the author of *Everything I Ever Wanted to Know I Learned in Kindergarten.* The story is of Greek philosopher Dr. Papaderos, who talks about his meaning of life and how he found it.

Dr. Papaderos, as a child in WWII, found a small piece of a mirror from a wrecked German motorcycle. He kept the mirror and used it as a toy to reflect light into dark places. As he got older, Dr.

Papaderos came to understand the mirror as a metaphor, that while he himself was not actually the source of the light that the mirror reflected, he could *be* light by spreading truth, understanding, and knowledge. Although he was but a fragment of the mirror himself, he could, by his light, shine in many dark places (including dark hearts of mankind). This was his meaning of life.

Debbie, a massage therapist, told me as she worked her magic on my arthritic neck and back, "We chase our role models, but really we need to be our own best role model." Like Dr. Papaderos, I too want to be a fragment of the mirror and shine light for others. I want to see the best in people and do my best for myself and others; I want to be the best version of me possible and be my own best role model.

THE NON-PATIENT

There Is No "Back to Normal"

Be careful of using the word "normal" around cancer patients, whether they call themselves a survivor or not.

THE FRUSTRATION OF NOT FEELING good is often heightened when illness or its side effects are no longer visible, as others often assume "normalcy" has returned. Tami, a breast cancer survivor who had a double mastectomy, has a favorite saying, "I don't look sick and you don't look stupid, yet here we are." Harsh, but on point.

As a person dealing with a chronic illness, it is exasperating when *looking* normal seems to equate to *being* normal. This dichotomy is common in the cancer world. It is often forgotten or unknown to those on the outside that while there is not necessarily a cast or a bandage as a reminder of an illness, there may still be mutating cells lying in wait to again ravage their hosts' body. The chronic condition and lasting side effects are not always gone just because the patient has completed treatment.

Anastasia told me that some of her most difficult issues came with the fact that she *did not* lose her hair. She found herself constantly explaining that she still had cancer and still took chemo pills every other day, leaving her just as sick as those who were bald.

There is always a "pass" for those who would not otherwise know a person was chronically ill, be it a stranger or someone on the very outer circle of one's life. Those people understandably see us for how we present; we all get that. It is the friends and family who actually know what's behind the false-normal of hair growth and normalized weight that the phrase "Now that you are *back to normal* ..." is like a knife to the heart.

Pity is not the goal; understanding is. We will never be normal again. Our new normal, as most of us refer to it, is where we are today and how we gauge our abilities moving forward. We cannot compare our current state to where we were prior to diagnosis; it's too painful and sometimes devastating to realize we may never have that normal again. The people we used to be are no longer with us as a result of the physical, mental, emotional, and spiritual upheaval we have endured. And while we can draw on our old self and spend time in reflection or even admiration of the people we once were, we will never be our old normal again. As patients, we must recognize and accept where we are now or we will go mad.

Yet having a new normal is not always bad. I have been surprised and impressed that every cancer patient I have talked to has, in at least one way, appreciated their new normal more than their pre-diagnosis normal.

Not one of us likes our diagnosis or anything that comes with it, but the change in ourselves, the innermost being of who we are is appreciated and understood and, in many ways, makes us grateful. Some even feel a sense of sorrow for those who have not had the opportunity to understand the perspective shift that comes with a chronic or terminal illness.

There will always be those who are chronically bitter and incurably angry or just flat-out ornery about their diagnosis; that's okay. Personally, I don't have the energy for that type of behavior. I have only so much energy—I see it as literally a handful (picture me cupping my hand as if holding water in it)—and I refuse to squander the precious resource by being a Negative Nelly. I have surrounded myself with positivity through my journey, which includes other patients who exude light and love and share the good they have found through their journey.

Each of us have moments of negativity, regardless of our appreciation for our new life. However, we have a choice as to whether we stay in the negative or move to the positive. As the Law of Attraction states, *focusing on positive or negative thoughts brings positive or negative experiences into a person's life*. I choose to put out positive energy and words, which in turn attracts like-minded, positive people. It's hard to stay in the realm of doom and gloom when you are surrounded by positivity.

Most cancer patients will never feel the same again, and some of us will never look the same. We are often plagued by lasting fatigue that knocks out our ability to be as physically active as we once were. Some of us remain on a barrage of medications that alter our moods, our physique, or our thoughts. We have scars and deformities from our fight, and implants where our original body parts were before. We will never be the same "normal" we once were.

So, in a nutshell, please stop hoping for your loved one to go *back to normal* ... and certainly never say that phrase to a patient.

Cure Is a Four-Letter Word

*Once you've had a cancer diagnosis, being "cured" may be
an unreachable goal. And the fear never goes away.*

"REMISSION IS A LESSON IN guarded optimism rather than magical
thinking," is a line I read from a blog post by Steve Jacob, a consultant for Baylor, Scott & White Health, who was describing remission,
and I appreciated it immediately.

The word "cure" is often misconstrued as "remission" and,
conversely, remission is often thought to mean cure. Unfortunately,
those words are mutually exclusive and can be painful when misunderstood or misused.

Remission is essentially classified as either partial or complete.
At its truest level, it means there is no evidence of active cancer at
the moment.

A cure, on the other hand, is defined as cancer never coming
back again. That is a pretty lofty statement, since there is always a
chance of relapse. Once diagnosed with cancer, being "cured" can
really only be used if the person reaches their death without ever
experiencing the cancer again. Therefore, "cure" is just too big a word
for most of us to feel comfortable with.

As a patient who has been told there is no cure for her disease,
the word remission feels like the heavens opened up and the angels
sang; it really doesn't get much better. Cure, however, feels like
a pipe dream, out of reach and inconceivable. Regardless of how
long a person has been in remission, we still hold our breath during
checkups and hear the whisper in our head: "Is it back?"

Before becoming fluent in the language of cancer, I thought cure and remission were interchangeable. Now I realize that remission is the only dream we have and cure lives somewhere in fantasy land. Many patients will go in and out of remission, some more than once during their journey, and each time they have to deal with the, "But weren't you cured?" question from family and friends.

Perhaps some of this responsibility for confusion lies with the patient, and we should use language that is less confusing and more accurate, such as No Evidence of Disease (NED); No Evidence of Active Disease (NEAD); and "dormant." A non-patient cannot be expected to understand what a sting the word "cure" can have.

Laughing in the Face of Cancer

Gallows humor is a healthy response for someone with cancer, no matter how dire their circumstances are. Facing disabilities—and even death—makes them targets for humorous possibilities.

"HUMOR IS IMPORTANT, BUT YOU are missing a lot if you only use humor to cope." This statement came from a man I know as Captain Obvious. He has a subtle, dry sense of humor, and to hear him say this was comical in and of itself. He is right though—while humor is important in dealing with illness, it is important not to sugarcoat everything.

That being said, many in my cancer group of friends have a twisted sense of humor about their disease. We seem to find irony and cynicism about our illnesses to be terribly funny. We are generally the only ones who think our humor is funny, however, and many on the outside of the diagnosis, including my husband, think it is morbid.

"I love the look on people's faces when I tell them, 'I have had three breasts removed.'" Susan had a double mastectomy and a complicated reconstruction that required the removal of one of her implanted breasts. Using her quick wit, she likes to drop this line and leave the recipient to ponder the statement; I fell into her trap when I first met her. Susan also apparently had the gift of singing in the recovery room following her mastectomy. She woke up singing a modified lyric from *The Wizard of Oz*: "Ding dong, the cancer's gone."

We cancer patients also tend to jokingly use our impending death as leverage, "I don't have much time you know!" or "You know I could die tomorrow ... seriously ..."—talk about awkward silence on the other end of that one.

We make jokes about the medicines we take, always referring to them as *drugs*. "I never did drugs until I got cancer," and "Who cares if marijuana isn't legal, what are they going to do, arrest me? I'm dying!"

We think it is funny to make jokes about how we already have cancer: "After all, what's the worst that could happen? I get cancer?"

My youngest son and I have used the same text message to each other over the years when we have gone a while without hearing from one another. Now that I am terminally ill, we think this particular banter is hysterical, while others find us macabre. He will text me with, "Are you dead?" and I will respond with, "Not yet!"

Michael, always the jokester, claims his testicular cancer, with subsequent orchiectomy (removal of his testicle) followed by the implantation of a prosthetic testicle, has given him a great bar trick: showing off his prosthetic testes. He will simply ask anyone in the bar if they would like to see his prosthetic testicle, then wait for their reaction when this statement sinks in. (Of course, he cannot really show off his prosthetic testicle—it is surgically implanted—he just wants to see how many people will say they want to see his testicles!)

We tend to find humor in the issues that happen to our bodies. The one I liked to tell about myself was regarding hair loss. No one really explains how the hair loss thing will go. I was thinking it would all fall out at once, like a tree in a comic strip that drops its leaves all at one shot, and then I would be bald. That is not at all the case. It is more like molting, when the feathers of a bird fall out a few at a time, some in clumps and some individually, leaving the bird looking more like a shaggy, pitiful creature rather than a gorgeous flying machine. I found it comical when the hair on my head started coming out in clumps. I called my youngest son over to my house, as Jody was out of town, and had him shave my head. But not before we got some good laughs as I literally pulled the hair from my scalp, leaving bald patches.

While this was entertaining for my son and I, the *real* funny story (which my husband is always amazed and perhaps a little mortified that I tell) is that the random molting process also happened to my "nether region." For whatever reason, only the pubic hair on my right side fell out, leaving me with the most interesting look for two weeks, until the left side finally caught up. I confided about my one-sided molting to my girlfriends one day at lunch. We hooted and hollered over this and had great laughs. A couple weeks later when I saw the same group of girlfriends, I told them that both the left and right sides were now equally bald. It was then that my friend Lisa, while nearly crying at the craziness of my hair story, admitted that she couldn't wait to tell her husband Mike that the rest of my hair fell out. I was aghast that she told Mike my story, but my friend Dawn also then sheepishly admitted she had told her husband about my hair loss. We all hooted some more at the ridiculousness of it.

One of the funniest stories I heard from other patients was from Pam regarding her breast cancer. She had a double mastectomy and decided not to do the reconstruction. Instead, she purchased "foobs" (fake boobs) to insert into her bras. As an avid swimmer, she was excited to start swimming again at her local community pool after her surgery. Her swimsuit, however, did not have built-in pockets to hold her new foobs. She bought some material and sewed the pockets in herself, happy with her accomplishment. She went to the pool on opening day with her son and grandson in tow, her swimsuit on, and her new foobs securely placed in their pockets. She enjoyed some time floating on her back, looking into the clear blue sky and smiling about how happy she was to be back in the pool. When she came back to an upright position, she noticed the pool was full of people smiling at her. Unbeknownst to Pam, the foobs had floated out of their pockets, up the V-neck of her suit and out into the pool. She laughs when she tells this story, saying, "Foobs—who needs 'em?"

Never Put off Anything on Your Bucket List

"Don't be afraid of death. Be afraid of the half-lived life."
—*Laird Hamilton*

I HAVE NO BUCKET LIST; at least no list that I have written down since being diagnosed. There are places I would like to see and things I would like to do, but they are just that, places and things, not burning desires.

I have lived a full life, being able to travel to fabulous places and having had incredible experiences. I have loved many and have been loved in return. I have watched my children grow up to become wonderful young men, and I have reconnected with God. Life is fabulous, and I am grateful for every day.

When I hit the point in my cancer journey where people would ask if I had a bucket list, I realized that list should already have been completed, as there was no energy to give toward anything outside of treatment. Those days of jetting around the world, climbing to the top of a mountain, or diving the Great Barrier Reef were over, at least until I got back on my feet. *If* I got back on my feet. From my perspective, those desires should have been met while I was healthy, not after I was diagnosed.

By the time a person hits the traditional end-of-life bucket-list stage, they generally can be so fatigued from fighting for their life, so exhausted from worry and fear, and so overwhelmed with the number of days they feel they may have left, a bucket list isn't always the top priority—friends and family are. The bucket list, left too late, can turn into more of a litany of "I wish I hads" and "Now I can nevers."

A bucket list should not be the last-ditch, end-of-life, grappling-to-accomplish-things list. A bucket list should be a continual, conscious effort to move forward by doing the things that make you happy and fulfilled, not a fleeting idea that comes when you realize your time on earth is short and you regret the things you did not do. During active cancer treatment, there is no time or energy for lists beyond doctors' appointments and treatment schedules.

Prior to being diagnosed, I did have a wish list of things I wanted to do, my "unfinished" goals. Perhaps it would be looked at as a "soft" bucket list, as it surely wasn't riddled with world-changing adventures. My list included learning to dance (waltz and salsa to be specific), getting back on a horse, river rafting, volunteering for the betterment of others, fly fishing, and playing the guitar. I had written those things down long before I was sick, while I was healthy and vibrant, and I started ticking them off one by one, regardless of how big or small, how silly or serious.

I did learn to waltz and salsa, among many other dances. I even tried belly dancing once, but it was not my cup of tea, which was unfortunate, as I really enjoyed the costumes and the sensuality of the dance. I relearned to ride a horse, I spent a summer river rafting, I picked up the guitar but never did anything further with it, and I returned to volunteering each week, which filled my soul with happiness. Accomplishing items on my list was self-gratifying and fulfilling.

As a cancer patient, it can be difficult to hear the words, "What's on your bucket list?" as the implication to someone with a life-threatening disease is that people must think the end is near. There can also be a lot of self-imposed pressure for this list to be magnanimous in order to be worthy. I think many non-patients are curious as to what people who are terminally ill think about regarding a bucket list. I asked the bold question to my cancer circle and the answers were widely varied.

Nikko enjoys the *thought* of a bucket list. For her, the idea of drifting out of her real life and into her bucket list of dreams brings her happiness. She is aware that many things on her list will never happen due to constraints of age, finances, time, and physical ability, but she enjoys the hope the fantasies bring her.

Mark recently ticked off rafting the Colorado River from his bucket list. He has four more items on his list, including climbing Machu Picchu in Peru. His brain cancer will likely not stop him from these accomplishments.

Chris wants to go on a dinosaur dig, and Anastasia marked

off auditioning for *America's Got Talent* as an accomplished item on her list.

Pam has no bucket list. She feels that she has had a fortunate life, and the most she wants to do now is revisit some favorite places with family to create new memories with them.

Denise feels generally the same as Pam. Her desire now is to have intentional relationships, sharing her time with those she loves, making sure they each know where their place is in her heart.

Jessica also simply wants to spend time with family and friends, watching her grandchildren grow, and traveling with her significant other.

When I asked Claire, who has stage 4 pancreatic cancer and is currently surviving with "over 100 tumors," how she felt about people asking her if she had a bucket list, she rolled her eyes, scoffed, and said, "That really pisses me off!" She explained that she has no bucket list because, "A. I don't have time for one with all the time it takes taking care of my health, and B. I don't have any energy to give to anything other than taking care of myself."

A bucket list can be a wonderful motivational tool. It can get you off the couch and out into the world. It can encourage you to learn a new language, try new foods, and explore new countries—a tool to help you achieve a life well lived. But it should be written when you are healthy and able. It should reflect your growth as a person and be a legacy to look back on, so this list should be thought about and cultivated throughout your life as your circumstances change.

Don't wait! Take the time to write down your desires, your dreams, your farfetched fantasies of the things you have always wanted to see, do, try, and accomplish—then pick one item and do it. Check it off and pick another item on the list. If you are lucky enough to complete them all, make a new list. There is no time to waste.

Reflections on Life Goals

*Cancer or any life-threatening illness changes what is normal
and what important goals look like—but it doesn't change
the essential person. It just takes them to a new place.*

WHEN I PAUSE TO REFLECT on where I was and where I am since
being diagnosed, the differences are staggering. I have reached my
two year "cancer-versary" of when I was diagnosed, and my former
self is almost unrecognizable.

I was a dancer and summertime outdoor enthusiast. I loved to
ride horses and river raft, hike, and travel. I was fit and healthy and
full of piss and vinegar. I would donate my extra time to helping
others in areas I felt passionate about. I spent years cooking each
week at a shelter for the homeless and served as a grief-group
facilitator for Mothers Against Drunk Drivers. I held the hands
of those dying in hospice care and was the reading mom at my
son's school. I was busy and energetic and fully immersed in my
community and my life.

My health is good again, from the standpoint of one with a
terminal illness. I currently have a head full of hair, weight on
my bones, and color to my face, but I am still lacking in stamina
and overall strength. I rarely dance now. I want to and I hope
to—dream about it actually—but grooving a bit in my own living
room is about all I have in me currently. My health can be fragile,
and being around large groups of people and in close physical
contact with them can actually be dangerous. There are times
when I become "neutropenic," which essentially means my white
blood cells (the ones that fight off infection) dump without any

warning or symptom, and I am left walking around without any white blood cells.

I am susceptible to colds, flu, and bacteria from food buffets and door handles. No different than anyone else, really, except those bugs to an immunocompromised individual can be especially lethal. Even fighting off the common cold is sometimes more than a person in that state can overcome.

Steve was in remission from esophageal cancer when he contracted E. coli, probably at a restaurant while on vacation with his wife. With his compromised immune system, he would never recover from that infection and would lose his hard-fought, years-long cancer battle to food poisoning. Others have been in remission, contracted a common cold, and passed away weeks later because their immune system could not shake what turned, for them, into a deadly virus.

As my health improves, I am trying to regain some semblance of my former self, become more active, and get back into shape. I find now, however, that my relationships are more important than my hobbies. And while I still want to be a part of my community and give back, I am doing it in a less visible way, more in the background where my contact with strangers is often more cyber and through the written word than face-to-face. I cannot control the health environments in my previous volunteer venues, therefore I have had to substitute those with safer choices.

This difference in my life is again reflective of a cancer shift, where the things, events, and hobbies that once trumped my relationships no longer do. I am learning to be okay with not being in as great of shape or as sociable as before in order to have the time and energy to cultivate and nurture the relationships that matter to me most.

Susan beautifully explained her cancer shift in a journal:

> *I have learned a lot in this journey. I have had to learn to accept my body not always doing what I want it to do. I am learning to accept the scars and changes to my body that treatment and surgeries have left behind. I don't get to choose, ultimately, how I will look as this journey continues. But I do get to choose how I feel.*

PART FOUR

Life Is Short ... for Everyone

Choosing how to live the rest of your life with however much time you have.

I'm the Lucky One: I Have Time to Get My S*** Together!

Cancer is a stark reminder that life is short. Learning to live in the moment may include taking action to "clear the decks" of unfinished business in your life.

THE BEAUTY, IF THERE IS one, in being told you have a terminal disease is that you can (theoretically) have the necessary conversations you feel need to happen while you are still here.

For me, I didn't reach out to my group of "long losts" until I was about eight months into my treatment and finishing up my trial drug regimen prior to moving into my in-patient chemotherapy. I reached out to three people.

Jody and I had only been married just over a year when I was diagnosed, and I had previously been single for many years. During my single life, I met and dated some amazing men. Obviously none of them worked out relationship-wise, but they were amazing nonetheless. In particular, there were three gentlemen I held dear long after our relationships ended. I reached out to them. I really had only one thing to say to them: I wanted them each to know I had always held them in the highest regard and felt fortunate to have had the time with them that I did. Essentially, I wanted to tell them I loved them.

When I tell people this story, I often get a perplexed look, as if I just crossed a line that no married woman should be telling another man (two of whom are also now married) that I loved them. It is unfortunate that a profession of love can be misconstrued as sex or desire. That simply was not the case. I loved these men for who they were and how they treated me; they were special people regardless of their gender and they deserved to know they were held in high esteem. I said my piece and was done. All three were surprised to hear from me and grateful that I reached out. These were restorative conversations. How many of us would be honored to hear that long after a split, someone still held us fondly in their thoughts? I would love to get that call! And so I would encourage everyone to have these types of conversations; perhaps everyone's lives would be better for hearing that they mattered to another person.

I also reached out to a few girlfriends from times gone by and reconnected, if only briefly, to let them know that they mattered to me and that while we may not have stayed connected, they were a positive light in my life. As with the three men, these women were all surprised and grateful I had taken the time to reach out.

The idea of getting my life in order before I die almost makes me chuckle; I wish I'd had the wisdom I have now long before I was diagnosed with cancer. There are many things to be done that I do not want to leave to my family to take care of, and quite honestly, there are some things I don't want anyone to "find." I am not a woman of great mystery, but some things I hold personal and private. For example, old photographs of me and others prior to marrying my husband. While those may not seem bad, they may be hurtful to Jody when I am gone. He may wonder what was so special that made me hang onto them after we were married. I might feel the same way if our roles were reversed, so I will make sure those are not around for him to find.

I am also working on the legalities of my life after death. I have my will and other legal papers wrapped up and am working on making sure I have my bank accounts and properties placed in someone else's name (not solely in mine), and I am generally doing all the things I should have done long before my diagnosis. I guess I thought I would live forever, or at least several more decades, and could get around to these things later. My later is now, and I'm finding a surprising amount of comfort in getting my s*** together!

My "Live" Funeral

I want a celebration of my life to be held
while I am still actually alive.

PART OF GETTING MY AFFAIRS in order was figuring out my funeral plans. This might seem macabre to some, but we all die, so isn't it better to get what you want? I realized, when talking to my friend Ray before he passed away, that I needed to figure out what I wanted done when I died.

Ray and I met on a flight to MD Anderson, a cancer hospital in Houston, Texas, where we both hoped that traveling to this health-care mecca would save our lives. Thus far it has worked for me, but it did not work for Ray.

He was a large man, towering over my five-foot-one-inch frame with his six-foot-five-inches, but he was frail and looked like cancer with his sunken eyes, inability to walk, and grimace of pain with every movement. He was, however, alive with a spark of life that everyone who encountered him could see. He was an instant friend.

Days before Ray passed, I was able to spend sixty seconds with him at his hospital bedside. Randomly, he told me, "'I Can Only Imagine' and 'Goodbye Friend' are my funeral songs." He also told me he could never quite understand the Book of Psalms in the Bible. This made me smile because I felt the same way.

"All those parables," he said. "What do they really mean?"

"I'm not sure," I told him.

It was a pretty random conversation, but obviously he had been thinking about something and felt he needed to say it. I learned, as I watched him decline through the months, that the closer one is to death, the less time they have for frivolous conversation. I left Ray's room and walked downstairs with his wife and told her about Ray's desired funeral songs.

"How do you know that?" she said to me. "You were only in there a minute."

Both songs were played at Ray's funeral. After his funeral, I decided I wanted to have a "live" funeral before I died. Jody thought this was morbid. My children, however, understood. I tried to explain to Jody it felt like an affront to think people would come to my funeral and say, "Wow, she was a great gal. Too bad I hadn't seen her in the past twenty years." To that I say, "Then why did you bother now?!"

I like the idea of a celebration of life, but I think it has somewhat missed the mark. I want to be at my celebration. I want to see my friends from decades gone by; the ones I went to high school with, the people I knew from the different cities I had lived in, and the people I know now. Why shouldn't the *alive* me be included in my celebration of life?

My celebration will include all my favorites: traditional turkey dinner with all the fixin's, especially the cranberry sauce that comes out of a can like a Jell-O mold, mountains of chocolate, fresh fruit, and cakes with many different frostings. The songs will be the ones memorable to me from disco, blues, Christian, and country.

My youngest son feels I should include the song, "Heaven Must be Missing an Angel." Not because he thinks his momma is an angel from heaven, but because it is a song on the *Charlie's Angels* soundtrack that was a favorite when my kids were growing up. When they were young, I would play that soundtrack over and over. When the "Heaven Must be Missing an Angel" song would play, we would do a little skit with hand movements to the line, "Your kiss, filled with tenderness." We would all simultaneously kiss our hand and blow the kiss away just after the word "kiss." This silly little gesture would make us all laugh like we had just heard the funniest joke. Those are great memories, and *that* is what I want at my funeral.

And, like Ray, I too want the song, "I Can Only Imagine." I am very spiritual and have a deep personal connection with that song; it doesn't hurt that it has a lyric in it about would you dance before Jesus. To that I say, "Yes!"

I would also like to have an open mic at my celebration, something we did at my dad's funeral. Of course, some of the people at Dad's service told sappy stories that made the whole room weep, but others told funny ones.

One of my dad's best buddies told a great story. He said, "I remember the day Fred took on a dare to ride his snowmobile across what he thought was a frozen lake. If he did it, I bought dinner. If he failed, he bought dinner. I let him sit there on that sled with the water up to his knees until I could get my camera out and take a picture. Fred bought dinner that night." I want to hear those types of fun memories from my friends. I want to laugh and cry with them, and to let them know they are loved by me. Before I die, I want to be able to interact with my friends. I would like to be able to help them understand that I am not afraid to die and to help make sure they each know how appreciative I am they were in my life.

The only snag I see with this plan is when to have my celebration. Jody has gotten on board with this idea and laughs with me now saying, "Yah, this is going to go over well, you have your live funeral and then carry on for another five years!" But what a good problem to have, I think.

I have run my live funeral idea past several of my "diagnosed" friends, and it has been met with resounding positivity. The general consensus is that we would rather see you and celebrate our lives with you while we are still alive. Don't hide from us or our impending death. We want you to celebrate our lives with us.

Not Afraid to Die

What do you say to a dying girl? Anything you want.

MY BOSS, DOUG, HAS SOMEWHAT of a lack-of-filter personality. While he is not a rude man, he is blunt. And the fact that he and I have worked together in a one-man (and one-woman) law firm for years makes our relationship an interesting one. He says what is on his mind, and I let it roll off my back. In all fairness, I too say what I want, and he in turn lets it roll off his back; a symbiotic relationship.

When I first told Doug about my diagnosis, he took a deep breath, leaned back in his chair, and made a gesture like a Catholic sign of the cross (touching his forehead, middle of his chest then each shoulder). He said, "Whew, sorry it's you but glad it's not me!" He then leaned forward in his chair and asked matter-of-factly, "Are you afraid to die?" I told him I didn't know yet as I hadn't had time to think about it.

We both laughed, thinking this was good banter. Doug's wife, however, upon learning of this, was not as enthusiastic about her husband's humor and worried about how it would sit with me. I appreciated her concern but appreciated his raw honesty more. All of us, in the deep recesses that we don't want to admit exist, feel the same way when someone else is diagnosed: we feel bad for them but are relieved it isn't us. This time around, I was the one who didn't dodge the bullet.

I Was Afraid, Initially

NATURALLY, IT TOOK A WHILE for my diagnosis to sink in, and when it did, I was initially terrified at the thought of dying. I knew that my spiritual life was in order, but I was still afraid. Some may say that's because my faith wasn't strong enough. I counter that by saying my free will was too strong. I had to learn to surrender, to give in to the knowledge of the finality to come, and accept that my disease would ultimately win. It wasn't about faith, it was about being content with knowing there will come a time when my fight is over. Knowing that

I will lose this war, not because I gave up or didn't try hard enough, but because it was my time; my lot in life.

There is a calmness about me, regardless of any visible emotional state I may be in. The calm I am referring to is internal. My heart no longer races when a bill doesn't get paid, and my palms don't get sweaty when I make a mistake at work. I am okay with the speeding ticket—I surely deserved it—and in the big scheme of things none of that really matters anyway. I have cancer. I have a terminal form of the disease, and no matter how I fill my life with things and events and people, or how hard I try, I will never outrun the inevitable. Giving into that knowledge has allowed me to fight my battle in a positive way with a happy heart. I will lose one day and that's okay because the reality is we all ultimately lose; all life is finite.

People squirm when they learn there is no cure for my disease. They will suggest that anything is possible, or I might be "the one" who defies the odds, or they throw the Hail Mary and remind me that "miracles happen." I don't think my death is looming around the next corner, and I *feel* I still have years left to live. But I am also a realist. I don't live in rainbow and unicorn land. I don't know when my time will come—no one does—but I now live my life free of that nonsensical worry, and I have never been happier.

If someone you love or care about has cancer, reach out to them to help them in the best way you know how. Find a way to let them know how you feel—your honest, heartfelt emotions for them and about their illness and what they have meant to you in your life. It will likely bring unexpected joy and peace to both of you.

Don't be afraid of going outside your comfort zone; you will be glad you did. I offer you this as a way to clean your own decks, while you can. Life is short for us all.

ACKNOWLEDGMENTS

I AM FOREVER GRATEFUL TO Jennifer Regner, my initial editor, and Maryanna Young of Aloha Publishing for coming along side me to help make this dream a reality.

A huge thank you to Kate, Nina, and Andrew at Mascot Publishing for believing in me, for fast-tracking this project and for all their work: true professionals.

To Lorna Partington Walsh who put the polishing edits on my manuscript—wow, can you make a story awesome! Thank you.

To all those who spoke with me about your cancer, once again I cannot thank you enough for your willingness to be open and tell your stories.

The talented Chris Taylor—friend, artist, and fellow warrior— thank you for painting all of the portraits used on the book's cover. And to those who agreed to have your portraits painted, thank you for letting me share your faces with the world.

Thank you to my family and friends, especially Michelle who lived the creation of this book daily with me and put up with me through the ups and downs of writing and my constant "It's almost done" comments. Who knew this "book thing" was going to be so tough?

A big thank you to Dorothy and Lisa for reading my drafts and giving me their honest opinions, which helped keep me going. And to Ethel for reading EVERYTHING I ever write – I love you! Lucy.

A big thank you to Epic Experience, the organization and the people: you truly helped me learn to live beyond cancer.

I am forever grateful to my husband, Jody, for sticking by me through my cancer journey, even when I didn't make it easy for him to do so.

To my boys and their significant others I say, "I love you to the moon and back."

And to my Mom, thank you for all the life lessons you have taught me.

And to every one of you who followed my journey and encouraged me to write something that might be helpful to people affected by cancer's touch, I love you all!

APPENDIX I
Cancer Terminology

As you begin your cancer journey, you may be baffled by the medical, biological, and anatomical jargon that gets thrown around. This glossary comprises words and terms that you may hear.

Benign
Refers to a tumor that is not cancerous. The tumor does not usually invade nearby tissue or spread to other parts of the body.

Biopsy
The removal of a small amount of tissue for examination under a microscope. Other tests can suggest that cancer is present, but only a biopsy can make a definite diagnosis.

Bone marrow
The soft, spongy tissue found in the center of large bones where blood cells are formed.

Bone marrow biopsy

In a bone marrow aspiration and biopsy, a doctor or nurse uses a thin needle to remove a small amount of liquid bone marrow, usually from a spot in the back of the hipbone (pelvis) or sternum. The second part of the procedure removes a small piece of bone tissue and the enclosed marrow.

Bone marrow transplant

A medical procedure in which diseased bone marrow is replaced by healthy bone marrow from a volunteer donor.

Cancer

A group of more than 100 different diseases that can begin almost anywhere in the body, characterized by abnormal cell growth and the ability to invade nearby tissues.

Cancer-related fatigue (CRF)

A subjective symptom of fatigue experienced by nearly all cancer patients. Fatigue is one of the most common and distressing side effects of cancer and its treatment. CRF is often more intense, more severe, and more distressing than the feeling of being tired, and it is less likely to be relieved with rest than fatigue that is experienced by a healthy person.

Cancer-versary

An important date in the life of anyone with a cancer diagnosis. Some refer to it as their date of diagnosis or their date of remission.

Carcinoma

Cancer that starts in skin or tissues that line the inside or cover the outside of internal organs.

Chemotherapy

The therapeutic use of chemical agents to treat disease, especially the administration of one or more cytotoxic drugs (drugs that inhibit or prevent the function of cells, primarily used to treat cancer) to destroy or inhibit the growth and division of malignant cells in the treatment of cancer.

Chronic

Refers to a disease or condition that persists, often slowly, over a long time.

Chronic myelogenous leukemia (CML)

Characterized by increased proliferation of the granulocytic cell line without the loss of their capacity to differentiate. It accounts for 20 percent of all types of leukemia affecting adults.

Clinical trial

A research study that tests new treatments and/or prevention methods to find out whether they are safe, effective, and possibly better than the current standard of care (the best known treatment).

CT or CAT Scan

A computed tomography (CT or CAT) scan allows doctors to see inside your body. It uses a combination of X-rays and a computer to create pictures of your organs, bones, and other tissues. It shows more detail than a regular X-ray. You can get a CT scan on any part of your body.

Cure

To fully restore health. This term is sometimes used when a person's cancer has not returned for at least five years after treatment. However, the concept of "cure" is difficult to apply to cancer because undetected cancer cells can sometimes remain in the body after treatment, causing the cancer to return later, called a recurrence. Recurrence after five years is still possible.

Fine needle aspiration (FNA)

A type of biopsy procedure. In fine needle aspiration, a thin needle is inserted into an area of abnormal-appearing tissue or body fluid with samples removed and tested.

Immunosuppressant

Drugs, agents, or anti-rejection medications that inhibit or prevent activity of the immune system.

Immunotherapy

A type of cancer treatment designed to boost the body's natural defenses to fight cancer. It uses materials made either by the body or in a laboratory to improve, target, or restore immune system function. It may also be called biologic therapy.

In situ

In place. Refers to cancer that has not spread to nearby tissue, also called non-invasive cancer.

Integrative medicine

A combination of medical treatments for cancer and complementary therapies to help manage the symptoms and side effects of cancer.

Invasive cancer

Cancer that has spread outside the layer of tissue in which it started and has the potential to grow into other tissues or parts of the body, also called infiltrating cancer.

Leukemia

A cancer of the blood. Leukemia begins when normal white blood cells change and grow uncontrollably.

Lymphatic system

A network of small vessels, ducts, and organs that carry fluid to and from the bloodstream and body tissues. Through the lymphatic system, cancer can spread to other parts of the body.

Lymphoma

A cancer of the lymphatic system. Lymphoma begins when cells in the lymph system change and grow uncontrollably. Sometimes a tumor is formed.

Malignant

Refers to a tumor that is cancerous. It may invade nearby healthy tissue or spread to other parts of the body.

Mantle cell lymphoma (MCL)

A rare form of non-Hodgkin lymphoma. A blood cancer that affects white blood cells and can spread to other organs in the body. MCL accounts for about 6 percent of adult non-Hodgkin lymphoma in the United States.

Mass

A lump in the body.

Metastasis

The spread of cancer from the place where the cancer began to another part of the body. Cancer cells can break away from the primary tumor and travel through the blood or the lymphatic system to the lymph nodes, brain, lungs, bones, liver, or other organs.

Neutrophils, Neutropenic

An unusually low number of cells called neutrophils. Neutrophils are cells in the immune system that attack bacteria and other organisms when they invade your body. Neutrophils are a type of white blood cell. Bone marrow creates these cells. If you have an unusually low number of neutrophils, you are neutropenic.

New Birthday

The date a person receives a stem cell transplant is referred to by patients as their "new" birthday.

No evidence of disease (NED)

When no sign of disease is seen.

No evidence of active disease (NEAD)

When no sign of disease is seen.

Non-Hodgkin lymphoma (NHL)

Cancer that originates in the lymphatic system, the disease-fighting network throughout the body.

Oncologist

A doctor who specializes in treating people with cancer. The five main types of oncologists are medical, surgical, radiation, gynecologic, and pediatric.

Palliative care

Palliative care is any form of treatment that concentrates on reducing a patient's symptoms or treatment side effects, improving quality of life, and supporting patients and their families. It may also be called supportive care.

Polyp

A growth of normal tissue that usually sticks out from the lining of an organ, such as the colon.

Precancerous

Refers to cells that have the potential to become cancerous. Also called premalignant.

Primary cancer

Describes the original cancer.

Prognosis

Chance of recovery; a prediction of the outcome of a disease.

Progression-free survival (PFS)

The length of time during and after treatment that the cancer does not grow or spread further. This term is often used in the context of scientific research.

Protocol (in clinical trials)

A formal, written action plan for how a clinical trial will be carried out. It states the goals and timeline of the study, who is eligible to participate, what treatments and tests will be given and how often, and what information will be gathered.

PET scan

A positron emission tomography (PET) scan is an imaging test that allows your doctor to check for diseases in your body. The scan uses a special dye containing radioactive tracers. These tracers are either swallowed, inhaled, or injected into a vein in your arm depending on what part of the body is being examined.

PICC line

A PICC (peripherally inserted central catheter) line is a thin, soft, long catheter (tube) that is inserted into a vein in the arm, leg, or neck. The tip of the catheter is positioned in a large vein that carries blood into the heart. The PICC line is used for long-term intravenous (IV) antibiotics, nutrition, or medications, and for blood draws.

Port or Port-a-Cath

A central venous catheter is a tube that goes into a vein in the chest and ends at the heart. Sometimes this type of catheter is attached to a device called a port that is placed under the skin. The port and catheter are put in place in a minor surgery. The catheter helps carry nutrients and medicine into the body. It will also be used to take blood when needed for blood tests.

Radiation therapy

The use of high-energy rays to damage cancer cells stopping them from growing and dividing. Like surgery, radiation therapy is a local treatment that affects cancer cells only in the treated area. Radiation can come from a machine (external radiation) or from a small container of radioactive material implanted directly into or near a tumor (internal radiation).

Recurrence

Cancer that has returned after a period during which the cancer could not be detected. "Local recurrence" means that the cancer has come back to the same general area where the original cancer was located. "Regional recurrence" refers to cancer that has come back in the lymph nodes or other tissues near the original cancer site, usually by direct spread. "Distant recurrence" refers to cancer that has come back and has spread to other parts of the body, usually by traveling through the lymph system or bloodstream.

Regimen

A treatment plan that includes expected treatments and procedures, medications and their doses, the schedule of treatments, and how long the treatment will last.

Rehabilitation

Services and resources that help a person with cancer obtain the best physical, social, psychological, and work-related functioning during and after cancer treatment.

Remission

The disappearance of the signs and symptoms of cancer but not necessarily the entire disease. The disappearance can be temporary or permanent.

Sarcoma

A cancer that develops in the tissues that support and connect the body, such as fat and muscle.

Secondary cancer

Describes either a new primary cancer (a different type of cancer) that develops after treatment for the first type of cancer, or cancer that has spread to other parts of the body from the place where it started (see entry for metastasis).

Standard of care

Care that experts agree or guidelines show is the most appropriate and/or effective for a specific type and stage of cancer.

Tumor

A mass formed when normal cells begin to change and grow uncontrollably. A tumor can be benign (noncancerous) or malignant (cancerous, meaning it can spread to other parts of the body). Also called a nodule or mass.

APPENDIX II

Tips and Reminders for the Patient

Important: The author of this book is not a physician or medical provider and has no clinical training. The suggestions in this section are merely from her own perspective and opinion. Consult your physician before beginning any type of exercise program or changing your diet.

Be kind to yourself. This is likely the most stressful personal time of your life.

Take advantage of palliative care options through your local clinic and hospital, such as acupuncture, massage, reflexology, counseling, and spiritual support. Many of these services are offered at reduced or no cost to the patient (and some to the family). Insurance may cover some options as well.

Remove toxicity from your life (set boundaries). This includes people. You are in no position to deal with toxic chemicals (cleaning agents, pesticides, etc.) or excess stress. Now is the time to purge these and focus on yourself.

SLEEP. Sleep is imperative and restorative. Rest often. Give into the urge to nap; it's okay and necessary for your body to heal and recover. And, when rested, things always look a little brighter.

Seek counseling. No matter how big or tough or otherwise impervious you have previously been to needing mental help, emotional support, or just encouragement, now is not the time to be stubborn. Cancer clinics and hospitals have social workers and spiritual guides who can assist in this area. None of us are preprogrammed to know how to deal with cancer.

Keep in mind, many cancer patients need anti-anxiety and antidepressant medications. It's okay. Do what you need to do. Do not feel ashamed or embarrassed. Take care of yourself.

Find support groups, either online or in person. In today's vast interconnected online world, there is sure to be a place where you can find someone with your exact diagnosis. You do not have to go through feeling alone; there are people out there going through the same thing—you may have to search for them, but they are there. Find them. Connect with them. This will become one of your only places where you can truly vent and open up in a safe forum without fear of hurting your friends and family.

Be honest with your friends and family. If your friends and family are not supporting you the way you need, tell them. This is about you. Do not feel like you will be hurting their feelings or stepping on toes. They want to help—they just may not know how.

Keep a visible calendar with your appointments and schedule. This way, your family and friends can see when you may need help (bringing a meal during a day you receive treatment or picking up your kids when you have a doctor's appointment). If they can see it they can easier know what you may need.

Set time limits for when you can receive visitors. Cancer is exhausting.

Let people know that you are only seeing people at specific times. Let your caregiver be the "bad cop" if you feel you cannot set these boundaries. I worried about being rude, but my husband understood this and would set limits for my time with others on my behalf.

Eat food and drink water. Food tastes mostly disgusting while you're going through treatment, but you must eat. Eat whatever works for you and worry about the consequences of unhealthy food choices after you are back on your feet. And drink water as if your life depends on it, because it does. Water will help flush the toxins out of your body. Drink, drink, drink.

Following treatment, continue to be kind to yourself. PTSD is very real for cancer patients; you will always wonder if it is back.

Cancer-related fatigue (CRF) is equally as real as PTSD. The fatigue is overwhelming at times and inexplicable. Educate yourself and your family about this. It will help save a lot of strife whenever you are suddenly exhausted.

Stay positive. There are great strides being made with cancer research and people are surviving longer with fewer toxic drugs than in previous years. A positive mental outlook is not only good for the mind but also good for the body. Cancer thrives in a stressed out, negative environment. Don't give it one.

Exercise. Walk during and after treatment, if you can. Force yourself to move, even if you are lying in bed. Lift your arms and legs, tighten your muscles, just move. It helps get the blood flowing and the muscles firing. Atrophy is very real when going through treatment because it is often impossible to exercise as you previously did.

Again, be kind to yourself. It's worth repeating! Cut yourself some slack. It is okay to feel bad, it is okay to not want to move, it is okay to feel hopeless. You can have those days, but then you must, for your own sake, keep going.

APPENDIX III

Tips and Reminders for the Non-Patient

Say prayers. Be respectful that not everyone wants to be prayed for. If you don't know someone's religious preference, offer words such as *light and love, positive vibes,* or *positive thoughts.*

Be helpful. Bring a meal, offer to clean house, or run errands.

Remember the caregiver—they are in the trenches of the illness without any of the attention. They need TLC as much as the patient.

Be patient. Fear of illness and death are real, for both those facing it and those not. Be both patient with and present for each other.

Set boundaries. Keep in mind boundaries are necessary for cancer patients when someone is not supportive in appropriate ways.

Remain sensitive, for years after diagnosis. Even many years after a diagnosis, it is important to remain sensitive to the patient; they still live every day with the trauma of having had cancer, its lasting effects, and the fear of its return.

Get counseling. Therapy is a great idea but is not for everyone. It can, however, be hurtful if a non-patient is not receptive to the idea. Talk about it with your loved one and be honest.

Relationships will change when touched by cancer. Be honest with each other, chances are you are both equally as concerned and frustrated.

Have real conversations. Save the cutesy "words of encouragement" for a T-shirt slogan; cancer patients need real conversations.

Be positive, but don't overdo it. It's great to be positive but a Pollyanna-esque, unrealistic, overly positive approach can leave the person who has been diagnosed exasperated. They know the reality of their situation—don't try to push it off with too much false "happy speak."

Patient's negativity is okay. Allow the patient to be mad, depressed, and feel self-pity. There is nothing wrong with any of these feelings, and it is healthy to acknowledge them.

Support systems are vital for patients. Assist in finding a support system for a cancer patient. Friends may be willing to listen, but they may not completely understand what the patient is feeling or going through. There are copious online groups available, including live chat group forums. There are also plenty of in-person support groups available.

Help the patient seek out palliative care through their cancer clinic, or work with a social worker or a counselor.

Find a way to contribute; it helps the patient and their loved ones feel more connected with others outside of treatment. There is always a need for volunteers in cancer clinics, and contributing can be in ways as simple as playing the piano in the clinic, baking cookies to have in the waiting room, or knitting hats for those going through chemo. And although not necessarily easy but truly worthy, get your dog certified as a comfort animal to visit with patients.

There are many different cancers. Remember, *pink* is not the only color of cancer, try to be considerate of that when addressing patients.

Please let us go when it is time.

No more "back to normal" talk. Appreciate your loved one's new normal; do not constantly refer to the way they "used to be."

Cancer is always traumatic. Keep in mind the cancer patient may never fully recover from their traumatic experience or behave the way they did pre-diagnosis.

APPENDIX IV
Resources and Further Information

The following resources are not endorsed by this author nor researched for their credibility. All numbers and URLs listed were those available at time of writing and may not be current. This is not an all-inclusive list.

- AIM at Melanoma, 916-706-0599: aimatmelanoma.org

- American Brain Tumor Association, 800-886-2282: abta.org

- American Cancer Society, 800-227-2345: cancer.org

- American Childhood Cancer Organization: acco.org

- American Lung Association, 800-586-4872: lung.org

- American Psychosocial Oncology Society, 866-276-7443: apos-society.org

- American Society of Clinical Oncology, 888-651-3038; www.asco.org

- Angel Flight American (assists with transporting patients), 918-749-8992: angelflight.com

- Association of Oncology Social Work (database to search for oncology social workers), 215-599-6093: aosw.org

- Bladder Cancer Advocacy Network, 888-901-2666: bcan.org

- breastcancer.org

- Cancer Care, 800-813-4673: cancercare.org

- cancer.com

- Cancer Hope Network, 800-552-4366: cancerhopenetwork.org

- Cancer Legal Resource Center, 866-843-2572: cancerlegalresources.org

- Cancer Research and Prevention Foundation, 800-227-2732: charitychoices.com

- Caring Bridge: caringbridge.org (free, personal, and private websites to connect family and friends during a health challenge)

- Caring Info, (National Hospice and Palliative Care), 800-658-8898: caringinfo.org

- Centers for Medicare and Medicaid Services, 800-633-4227: cms.gov

- Center for Mind-Body Medicine, 202-966-7338: cmbm.org

- Children's Cause for Cancer Advocacy, 202-336-8374: childrenscause.org

- Chronic Disease Fund (financial assistance), 972-608-7141: mygooddays.org

- clinicaltrials.gov (referral for clinical trials)

- Colorectal Cancer Alliance, 877-422-2030: ccalliance.org

- Co-Pay Relief Program (financial assistance), 866-512-3861: copays.org

- Corporate Angel Network (transportation assistance), 914-328-1313: corpangelnetwork.org

- Emergingmed (to speak with a clinical trial specialist), 877-601-8601: app.emergingmed.com

- Family Caregiver Alliance, 800-445-8106: caregiver.org

- Family Reach (financial assistance), 973-394-1414: familyreach.org

- Fight Colorectal Cancer, 877-427-2111: fightcolorectalcancer.org

- Health Resources and Services Administration (resource for healthcare facilities that provide free or reduced-cost case), 800-638-0742: hrsa.gov

- HealthWell Foundation (financial assistance), 800-675-8416: healthwellfoundation.org

- Imaginary Friend Society (videos for children about cancer): team.curethekids.org

- Inflammatory Breast Cancer Research Foundation, 877-786-7422: ibcresearch.org

- Intercultural Cancer Council (Baylor College of Medicine), 713-798-4617: agable.net

- International Myeloma Foundation, 800-452-2873; myeloma.org

- International Waldenstrom's Macroglobulinemia Foundation, 941-927-4963: iwmf.com

- Joe's House (resource for lodging near treatment centers), 877-563-7468: joeshouse.org

- Kidney Cancer Association, 800-850-9132; kidneycancer.org

- Livestrong, 855-220-7777: livestrong.com

- Leukemia and Lymphoma Society, 800-955-4572: lls.org

- Living Beyond Breast Cancer, 888-742-5222: lbbc.org

- Lung Cancer Alliance, 800-298-2436: lungcanceralliance.org

- LUNGevity Foundation, 312-407-6100: lungevity.org

- Lymphoma Research Foundation, 800-500-9976: lymphoma.org

- Melanoma Research Foundation, 800-673-1290: melanoma.org

- Men Against Breast Cancer, 866-547-6222: menagainstbreastcancer.org

- MetaCancer Foundation, Inc.: metacancer.org

- Multiple Myeloma Research Foundation, 203-229-0464: themmrf.org

- mylifeline.org (blogs, online support)

- National Brain Tumor Society, 800-770-8287: braintumor.org

- National Breast Cancer Coalition, 800-622-2838: breastcancerdeadline2020.org

- National Cancer Institute, 800-422-6237: cancer.gov

- National Cervical Cancer Coalition, 800-685-5531: nccc-online.org

- National Children's Cancer Society, 314-241-1600: thenccs.org

- National Coalition for Cancer Survivorship, 888-650-9127: canceradvocacy.org

- National Hospice and Palliative Care Organization, 800-658-8898: nhpco.org

- National Lymphedema Network, 800-541-3259: lymphnet.org

- National Marrow Donor Program, 800-627-7692: bethematch.org

- National Ovarian Cancer Coalition, 888-682-7426: ovarian.org

- National Patient Travel Center (flight assistance for treatment or second opinion), 800-296-1217: rarediseases.org

- Native American Cancer Research, 800-537-8295: natamcancer.org

- NeedyMeds (financial assistance), 978-865-4115: needymeds.org

- Nueva Vida, 202-223-9100: nueva-vida.org

- Office of Minority Health, 800-444-6472: minorityhealth.hhs.gov

- Oncolink (culturally specific resources), 215-349-8895: oncolink.org

- Oral Cancer Foundation, 949-646-8000: oralcancerfoundation.org

- Ovarian Cancer National Alliance, 866-399-6262: ocrahope.org

- Pancreatic Cancer Action Network, 877-272-6226: pancan.org

- Partnership for Prescription Assistance, 888-477-2669: pparx.org

- Patient Access Network Foundation (financial assistance), 866-316-7263: panfoundation.org

- Patient Advocate Foundation, 800-532-5274: patientadvocate.org

- Patient Services, Inc. (PSI) (financial assistance), 800-366-7741: patientservicesinc.org

- Prostate Cancer Foundation, 800-757-2873: pcf.org

- The Prostate Net, 888-477-6753: theprostatenet.org

- Rosalynn Carter Institute for Caregiving, 229-928-1234: rosalynncarter.org

- Sisters Network, 866-781-1808: sistersnetworkinc.org

- Skin Cancer Foundation, 212-725-5176: skincancer.org

- Social Security Administration (financial support information), 800-772-1213: ssa.gov

- State Health Insurance Assistance Program (SHIP), 800-633-4227: medicare.gov

- Survivorship A to Z: survivorshipatoz.org

- Support for People with Oral and Head and Neck Cancer, 800-377-0928: spohnc.org

- Susan G. Komen Breast Cancer Foundation, 877-465-6636: komen.org

- Thyroid Cancer Survivor's Association, 877-588-7904: thyca.org

- Together RX Access (medication assistance), 800-444-4106: needhelppayingbills.com

- The Ulman Cancer Fund for Young Adults, 888-393-3863: ulmanfoundation.org

- United Way (financial assistance), 211: unitedway.org

- Uniting Against Lung Cancer, 212-627-5500: lungcancerresearchfoundation.org

- US TOO International Prostate Cancer Education & Support Network, 800-808-7866: ustoo.org

- Vital Options International, 818-508-5657: vitaloptions.org

- WomanLab: womanlab.org

- Young Survival Coalition, 877-972-1011: youngsurvival.org

- Zero—The Project to End Prostate Cancer, 888-245-9455: zerocancer.org

APPENDIX V
Cancer Support Colors

READ MORE ABOUT THESE COLORS at www.choosehope.com, which is an online shopping site where you can buy cancer-awareness merchandise designed and made by and for cancer survivors.

- All cancers – multicolored
- All cancers – lavender
- Appendix cancer – amber
- Bladder cancer – marigold/blue/purple
- Brain cancer – grey
- Breast cancer – pink
- Carcinoid cancer – zebra stripe
- Cervical cancer – teal/white
- Childhood cancer – gold

- Colon cancer – dark blue
- Esophageal cancer – periwinkle
- Gallbladder/bile duct cancer – Kelly green
- Head and neck cancer – burgundy/ivory
- Hodgkin lymphoma – violet
- Kidney cancer – orange
- Leiomyosarcoma – purple
- Leukemia – orange
- Liver cancer – emerald green
- Lung cancer – white
- Lymphoma – lime green
- Melanoma – black
- Multiple myeloma – burgundy
- Ovarian cancer –teal
- Pancreatic cancer – purple
- Prostate cancer – light blue
- Sarcoma/bone cancer – yellow
- Stomach cancer – periwinkle
- Testicular cancer – orchid
- Thyroid cancer – teal/pink/blue
- Uterine cancer – peach
- Honors caregivers – plum

REFERENCES

1. Beauty through the Beast, "50 Percent of Couples Break up During a Cancer Diagnosis," December 20, 2015, https://medium.com/@CancerBTTB/50-percent-of-couples-break-up-during-a-cancer-diagnosis-29133893975f

2. Ibid.

3. Metavivor, Historic Breast Cancer Research, Support and Awareness, https://www.metavivor.org/research/

4. Kathy LaTour, "Post-Cancer Fatigue: The Invisible Wound," August 3, 2018, www.curetoday.com/printer?url=publications/heal/2018/summer-2018/postcancer-fatigue-the-invisible-wound.